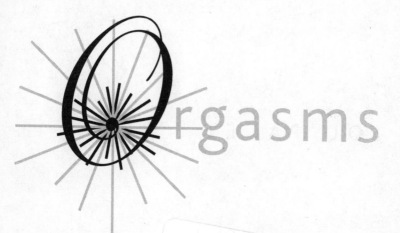

Orgasms

LOU PAGET

Also by Lou Paget

How to Be a Great Lover

How to Give Her Absolute Pleasure

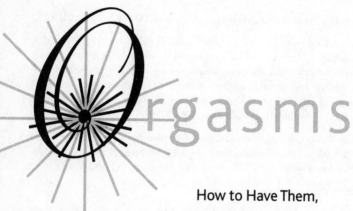

Orgasms

How to Have Them,
Give Them, and
Keep Them Coming

Broadway Books   New York

BROADWAY

Broadway Books titles may be purchased for business or promotional use or for special sales. For information, please write to: Special Markets Department, Random House, Inc., 1745 Broadway, New York, NY 10019.

PRINTED IN THE UNITED STATES OF AMERICA

BROADWAY BOOKS and its logo, a letter B bisected on the diagonal, are trademarks of Random House, Inc.

Visit our website at www.broadwaybooks.com

First trade paperback edition published 2005

Book design by Ralph Fowler

The Library of Congress has cataloged the hardcover edition as:
Paget, Lou
The big O, orgasms : how to have them, give them, and keep them coming / Lou Paget.
        p.   cm.
Includes bibliographical references.
1. Sex instruction. 2. Sex. 3. Orgasm. I. Title.
HQ31 .P24 2001
631.9'6—dc21   00-069917

ISBN 0-7679-0754-X

10   9   8

This book was written to inform, educate, and expand the awareness of its readers. While the techniques and products mentioned in this book work well for some people, they may not be appropriate for you. Be aware that it is your responsibility to know your body and that of your partner. This book talks about sex acts that are illegal in some states. Know your state's laws about sex, and if you choose to break them you do so at your own risk. This book makes no representation as, or as a substitute for, relationship counseling.

No one involved in the writing or publishing of this book is a physician, mental health professional, or licensed sex therapist, although members of those professions have been consulted on certain issues. Consult with a physician if you have any condition that precludes strenuous or sexually exciting activity. Further consult a physician or AASECT certified sex therapist before attempting any sexual act that you are unfamiliar with, or do so at your own risk.

Neither Lou Paget nor Broadway Books nor any of their associates shall be liable or responsible to any person or entity for any loss, damage, injury, or ailment caused, or alleged to be caused, directly or indirectly, by the information or lack of information contained in this book.

To all those who quest for
accurate information in the arena of human sexuality.
And for everyone who knows there can be
greater possibility and future in their own sexuality.

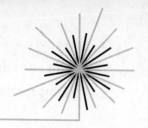

Contents

Acknowledgments   ix

CHAPTER ONE
The Big O   1

CHAPTER TWO
Debunking the Myths   11

CHAPTER THREE
The Physical Side of Orgasms   28
The Body's Responses

CHAPTER FOUR
Clearing Your Head   53
The Mental Side of Orgasms

CHAPTER FIVE

The Female Orgasm 69
Going for the Unexpected

CHAPTER SIX

The Male Orgasm 118
*How to Get the Most from
the Tools You've Got*

CHAPTER SEVEN

Medical Concerns That 148
Impact Sexuality

CHAPTER EIGHT

The Beauty of Enhancers 181

CHAPTER NINE

Sex and the Spirit 209

A Final Note 239

Appendix One
Sexually Transmitted Diseases (STDs) 240

Appendix Two
Resources: Where You Can Get the Toys 247

Bibliography 256

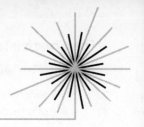

Acknowledgments

T ruly one of the best parts of writing a book is doing these pages . . .

The Support Team

As always some of my biggest and strongest has come from the ladies in my family: Dede, Katerena, Sherry, Lisa, Michelle, and Carolynn.

Jay Rosen, Frankly Speaking, Inc., marketing director, my business right hand. And he's great on the phone.

To all who have been there through yet another tour of duty: Jessica Kalkin, Bernard Spigner, Maura McAniff, Kendra King, Raymond Davi, Bryce Britton, Priscilla Wallace, Sandra Beck, Alan Cochran, Christine Hildebrand, Nance Mitchell, Morley Winnick, Eileen Michaels, Mark Charbonneau, Lilianna and Ali Moradi, Craig Dellio, Ron Ireland, Patrick Boyd, Flint Nelson, Paul Drill, Elaine Wilkes, Gwinn Ioka, Piper Dano, Matthew Davidge, Rhonda Britten, Rebecca Clemons.

The Creative Team

Billie Fitzpatrick: We did it again. And indeed the e-mails were equally as good this time around. Gretchen: for your patience through number 3.

Debra Goldstein: Dream agent, and so much more; and her support team Steven and Bodhi.

Lauren Marino: The book's Executive Producer, who sees it all and guides through the minefields.

Cate Tynan, assistant editor; Liz DeRidder, copyeditor; "J" the illustrator; Umi Kenyon the graphic artist for the cover; and Wanda Knight, who keeps those books coming.

Mary Anne Naples and Mark Roy at Creative Culture, Chandler Crawford for all the international sales, and all at Broadway Books.

The Research and Development Team

Penelope Hitchcock, D.V.M., Beverly Whipple, Ph.D., Patti Britton, Ph.D., Sherri J. Tenpenny, D.O., Gary Richwald, M.D., Joseph C. Wood, M.D., Stephen Sacks, M.D., Mitchell Tepper, Ph.D., Bernie Zilbergeld, Ph.D, Bryce Britton, M.S., Jacquie Brandwynne, Dennis Paradise, Dan and Shay Martin, Mark Fishman, and Jules S. Black, M.B., B.S.

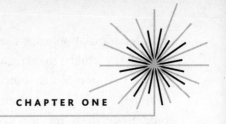

CHAPTER ONE

The Big O

The Ultimate Buffet

Doing sexuality seminars, I receive a lot of interesting, sometimes ludicrous questions about sex, specifically about orgasms. But the questions that most intrigue me are those that speak to men's and women's uncertainty about orgasms. I remember one woman in particular who had been recently widowed after a twenty-nine-year marriage. She said to me, "I don't know if I've ever had an orgasm. I think I have, but I'm not sure. How can I be sure?" This same feeling was echoed by a man who said that his girlfriend was convinced that she had had an orgasm, but he felt sure that she hadn't.

How can we be so uncertain about something so big? That's one of the questions I want to answer in this book.

Recently a French gentleman I know asked how it was possible for me to still be objective and open to sex after eight years of doing research, listening to hundreds and hundreds of stories, and reading countless books about sex. He thought my perception of sex must be "deformed" (give him a little room for translation error here). When I asked him why he thought my ability to perceive would be deformed, he explained that one of his companies had manufactured sound equipment and he had to train himself to know everything he could about these musical systems. As a result, he could no longer listen to music, all he would hear were the distortions of a system or equipment. "Ahh," I said. "There's a big difference. With music equipment, you know exactly how things should sound. With sex, there is no 'exactly as it should be.' Thank God!"

I want to be very clear that I see this book as one of possibility, not shoulds or should nots. What I mean is that everyone should be able to enter into a sexual situation with excitement, anticipation, and a sense that they may discover something new about themselves or their partner's likes and dislikes. No one should have to enter a sexual situation with fear or insecurity or the sense that they "should" be doing something they're not or "shouldn't" try something new or different. Heaven knows we have had plenty of messages of what we are supposed to be doing or feeling in the arena of sexuality. The fact is, in all the time that I have been doing the sexuality seminars, one of my strongest observations is the vast and wide continuum on which women and men experience sexual pleasure. There seems to be a limitless potential to what one can try, which in turn gives us a universe of possibilities to explore. I refer to this phenomenon as the ultimate buffet. Sometimes you may only want to sample an hors d'oeuvre, other times you might find yourself reaching for good old-fashioned comfort food, and then on occasion, you just might want a full-course meal, entrée included.

This book is about having the options to try. Think of sex

this way: Being intimate is like dancing. You kind of know where you are going, but you don't do the same step every time. You want a variety of moves that flow for you. As one man from a seminar said to me, "I know I want to have two or three things I do really well, and to know that they work for both of us."

If you've come to *Orgasms* after reading my two other books, you might have a question: How could there be more information about sex, specifically orgasms, that wasn't covered in the men's and women's books? Valid question. At first, I didn't think there could be more information—sure, a few details, but I couldn't yet imagine what else was out there related to orgasms that I hadn't already covered. Surprise! I discovered that there was a lot more to learn.

If you haven't yet read *How to Be a Great Lover* or *How to Give Her Absolute Pleasure* then not only will you learn all there is to know about orgasms, you'll learn that I see sex not as a performance experience with orgasm as its ultimate goal, but instead as a wide, meandering avenue toward pleasure— in whatever form you desire. An orgasm, of course, is a wonderful, satisfying state, but it should not be held up as the sole goal that drives your sexual experience.

As you may recall, during the 1980s, Americans seemed to be all about conspicuous consumption and amassing as many material goods as possible. Well, our attitude about sex and sexual experiences suffered from the same bonfire-of-the-vanities performance attitude, which dictated that you had to perform and amass extraordinary experiences. There were fairly set (predetermined) types of experiences that qualified as extraordinary, such as the multiple orgasm, which was rarely defined but always expected to occur. And what about the blitz on simultaneous orgasms? This hype had couples believing that if only they did X, Y, Z they'd discover the bliss of coming together every time they had sex! Fortunately, as we've shed or at least begun to question this consumption-oriented attitude, we as a culture have also begun to look at what makes us comfortable in all areas of our lives, including sex. The attitude has become more about making it simple, and my goal with *Orgasms* is to make this information smart, simple, and fun for you.

What I have also discovered in my research is the potential for a much broader range of orgasmic experiences than I had imagined. Not only does *Orgasms* assemble the most up-to-date information about orgasms for men and women, it also delivers it to you in a way that you can read alone or together as a couple, sharing details and experiences.

Now a small caveat here: A pox on anyone who tries to tell their partner they have a problem or are lacking technical skill or sensuality or do not experience one form of orgasm or another.

Before you get into the body of the information in the chapters that follow, I'll tell you a few reasons why I feel we should know more about orgasms. First, women and men experience orgasms very differently. Whereas men can experience an orgasm in up to seven different ways, women can experience orgasms in up to ten different ways! Have you ever heard of a mouth orgasm? A zone orgasm? Breast orgasms? Both sexes can and do experience all of these types. The second factor complicating orgasm information is the very physiological fact that men and women have very different sexual arousal cycles. From the starting gate, a couple trying to coordinate orgasms simultaneously generally faces very normal physiological challenges.

HISTORICAL AND HYSTERICAL FACTS	Throughout the ages, people have referred to sex in many different ways. Try these on for size:

- Come in and recognize her again (attributed to Louis XV)
- Fling one's spear into the future (Franz Liszt)
- Long conversation
- Disrespect for my person
- Tool (Lord Byron)
- Swive (Elizabeth I)
- Be overcome with sympathy
- Feel like a woman

The good news is that with the following information, you will have much more insight into your own body, your partner's, and orgasms in general. This book will give you awareness and permission to have an orgasm, seek one out—in whatever form you desire—and even choose not to have one, should that be your preference.

Although this book stands on its own in terms of complete information, you can also use it as a companion to the first two books. The way I like to think about the three books is that the first one is hers, the second one is his, and the third is for both of you, together. Readers already familiar with my work will recognize some techniques, including such now infamous manual sex techniques as Ode to Bryan, and oral techniques, including the Ring and Seal. I repeat them here for new readers and in the event you need a refresher. For new readers, welcome, and bear in mind that these oral and manual techniques are just the tip of the proverbial iceberg. In other words, if these techniques work for you and your partner, you can further add to your sexual repertoire with the information in the other two books.

My feeling about women and their sexuality is that they are entitled to accurate, respectful, fun information that works for them. I echo that sentiment for men and add further that if women have cultural permission to not know about sex, then men should be afforded that same prerogative. Men don't have cultural permission to not know about sex, and hence they often receive or infer inaccurate information about their own or women's bodies.

HISTORICAL AND HYSTERICAL FACTS	The most active time for sex in the United States is 11 P.M., especially on weekends.

The majority of couples I meet want to keep their sexual relationships alive and new. Yet they know that, regardless of age, if they've been together five months, five years, or twenty-five years, sex will gradually lose the newness of that thrilling beginning. I hope this book will provide couples with some options and ideas to retain or infuse their sex lives with freshness and energy. With this in mind, I've tried to capture techniques that will help either launch new couples or rejuvenate those who have been together for a while.

One of the recent trends I've noticed in giving my sexuality seminars is the growing curiosity and willingness to experiment—be it with sexual toys or sexual styles. Often, once women and men experiment with a particular toy—the Rabbit Pearl, for example—they begin to incorporate it into their sex lives. They may not do this all the time—just when they want to heighten the variety factor.

Other cutting-edge information included in the book comes from brand-new research in the area of the physiological sexual responses in men and women. Specifically, researchers can now trace—with tremendous accuracy—the neural and muscular pathways orgasms follow in the body. With this information, we can now know where the nerves are on which these specific responses travel, and hence, that gives us a better ability to create and enhance orgasmic responses.

Such prescription drugs as Viagra have certainly opened the doors further. It's interesting to know how scientists stumbled on Viagra's orgasm application. Originally, it had been developed as a heart medication. When researchers had finished their clinical trials, they found that men in the study were not returning their trial samples. What they later discovered was that these men were having erections and had become potent for the first time in years. No way were they going to give back the sample drug! Pfizer hit a home run with that accident.

In the area of women's orgasms, we have seen "orgasm trends" come and go. First, there was unassailable predominance of the clitoral orgasm, then it became the quest for a G-spot orgasm, and before women had time to catch their breath, they were told that *all* women experience ejaculation when they orgasm. While all these orgasms can occur in women and have been known to give certain women tremendous sexual pleasure, they are not universal truths. I hold the American media and the adult pornography industry responsible for establishing false and unrealistic expectations. In most cases these forces are not acting out of meanness or ill intent, rather, they are simply not as up-to-date or aware of the information as they could be.

| **HISTORICAL AND HYSTERICAL FACTS** | According to a recent report in the *New England Journal of Medicine*, women are 30 percent more sexually active during a full moon. |

How is a woman to know what's true, partially true, or not at all true because a certain fact may have been taken out of context?! In chapter 2 I will go into more depth about just how certain myths about sexuality impact us on a daily basis.

In chapter 3 I describe the details of the physical side of orgasms—how your sexual organs are affected, as well as the rest of your body. I have included diagrams so you can orient yourself and your partner. Again, you will see that men and women differ here. With this information, you and your partner will have more knowledge and awareness of your differences and similarities. I've also included information on the most recent medications that impact—both positively and negatively—sexuality and the ability to orgasm. As always, I have taken into consideration factors such as age, physiological condition, and those ever-changing emotional conditions that affect your ability to enjoy sex.

Sex is a multidimensional experience: it is as much about the body as it is about the mind. Have you ever felt that your body wants to let go but your mind gets in the way? In chapter 4 I address the mental side of orgasms. How do our attitudes or expectations or fears get in the way of our pleasure? I'm an unrepentant believer in the attitude that allows you to be as free to seek as much pleasure as possible—in whatever way makes you comfortable—as long as it is safe—meaning you use methods to prevent unwanted pregnancy or the spread of disease. I'm not proposing that you run willy-nilly in the pursuit of just anything, but rather that you simply break down self-imposed barriers to pleasure. This alone can be a powerful force. Sex and specifically orgasms can make you feel vital, promote inner self-esteem, and give you more energy. If you share this energy with your partner, who knows the limits of your intimacy and pleasure! Why would you want to prevent this?

Naturally, the heart and soul of *Orgasms* are the two chapters that gather the latest information on the types and techniques of orgasms for women and men. In chapters 5 and 6 I open the lid on the vast reservoir of new information that has yet to reach the public. I describe information and positions that are the best for certain types of orgasms, as well as ways to adjust what you already know.

The next two chapters cover the medical issues related to orgasms (or what gets in the way of orgasms) and the enhancers that increase sensation and ways in which to access pleasure, including aphrodisiacs, massage techniques, and lubricants.

Saving the best for last, in chapter 9 I offer some ideas on how to make your sexual experience with your lover more of a spiritual experience. I describe my version of Tantra, culling information from the most exotic and ascetic of sources. You will learn ancient Eastern techniques for prolonging erection, controlling ejaculation, and extending the length and intensity of your orgasm. Interested in a cross-cultural visit?

This book is for you and your partner to share, read together, and most importantly to have fun. The information gathered is real, accurate, and meant to widen your horizons, pique your curiosity, or whet your appetite. Enjoy!

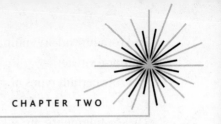

CHAPTER TWO

Debunking the Myths

The Myths

This chapter does just what it says: I expose the misinformation in the popular imagination regarding orgasms. Literally hundreds of myths still exist, getting in the way of having or enjoying an orgasm. Consider these particular myths:

- ➤ Simultaneous orgasms are more satisfactory than those experienced separately.
- ➤ Simultaneous orgasms are necessary for sexual compatibility in marriage.
- ➤ The best health is enjoyed by those who abstain from sex.
- ➤ A woman's repeated sexual experience with one man may leave a mark on a child later fathered by a different man.
- ➤ All women can orgasm during vaginal intercourse.

> Women who are multiorgasmic are of lower moral virtue.
> Only certain types of orgasms "really count."

These statements are all patently false, and in that way, misleading. Some are based on outdated scientific information that was later disproven, and others derive from religious belief that has a didactic if not repressive purpose. Another myth: Only men ejaculate. Nothing could be further from the truth! Many women, when they are aroused, will discharge fluid. This fluid is not urine; its source is the paraurethral glands on either side of the urethra. Hence the common assumption that it is urine.

SECRET FROM LOU'S ARCHIVES

According to sexologist Helen Fisher, "the female sex drive is more flexible: hence women have a greater tendency toward bisexuality. The feminine libido is also more intense (but less constant), embedded in a broader emotional and social context, and just as durable across the life course."

According to Dr. Beverly Whipple, who along with researchers Alice Kahn Ladas and John D. Perry named the G-spot, another myth associated with female ejaculation is that it occurs only with G-spot stimulation. Again not true. Some women ejaculate fluid when they get aroused, while others say they have never experienced ejaculation. There are still other women who realize that in fact they have ejaculated only after they hear confirmation that such a thing exists.

One woman in a seminar reported such a story about female ejaculation. She explained that she and her boyfriend were away on vacation staying in a "fancy hotel in London." One time, during sex, she was on top of him while he was giving her oral sex. She was getting more and more aroused, and getting closer and closer to climaxing, when her boyfriend gently pushed her away, claiming that she had just peed on him. Mortified, she ran to the bathroom. Needless to say, that ended their romantic moment.

Later, after they'd returned to New York, she'd wondered about the episode, not believing that she had actually urinated. When she came to one of my seminars and learned about female ejaculation, she had a "eureka!" moment. "Oh my God," she exclaimed. "That's what happened in London!" She had been so aroused and stimulated that her glands released the fluid. Relieved and no longer ashamed, she couldn't wait to go home and tell her boyfriend.

SECRET FROM LOU'S ARCHIVES

Freud was one of the first scientists to bring female orgasms public attention. Unfortunately, he claimed that only a vaginal orgasm is a "mature" orgasm.

This woman is not alone in such misconceptions about orgasms and our bodies. How many of the statements from the list above have you heard before and perhaps taken as truth? Is it obvious that these statements are outdated, half true, or abjectly false? How does one tell the difference or learn to distinguish?

Let's look at some myths more closely:

> If a woman doesn't have an orgasm before her first period, she may never be able to have one. False. There is no established age at which a woman experiences her first orgasm. Nor is there any age when it's not possible. About 23 percent of women experience their first orgasm by age fifteen and 90 percent by age thirty-five. These figures include orgasm from masturbation, a partner's manual and/or oral stimulation of the genitals, nocturnal dreams, and fantasy.

> A man has to have an erection in order to orgasm. False. Men can have what is called a "softgasm," which is an orgasm and ejaculation without an erection.

> Women who are menopausal are not interested in sex. False. The impact of menopause will often require adjustments to a couple's lovemaking, but in no way heralds the end of interest. No doubt, this myth is related to the passé idea that sex should only take place for procreation.

> One stops being sexual after a certain age. False. According to Drs. Milsten and Slowinski, a review of the data from Masters and Johnson Institute suggests that senior citizens have a very strong interest in sex. The oldest couple treated was a ninety-three-year-old man and his eighty-eight-year-old wife. Age is only a number.

> Men are always ready for sex. False. Just as women need foreplay to get relaxed and aroused, men too need foreplay and can't be expected to perform as if on cue.

➤ Masturbation causes impotence. False. This myth was perhaps dreamed up in Rome, to try and control the urges of some frisky members of the flock. There is no physiological, emotional, or spiritual link between masturbation and impotence.

➤ "Blue balls" makes you impotent. False. The blood engorgement of the scrotal testicle area may become sore and tender, but certainly not blue. As one man pointed out, "I mean let's get serious. Most men have a pretty good idea of how to take care of the problem themselves, and the balls don't actually turn blue anyway." Hard and hot, yes; blue, no.

SECRET FROM LOU'S ARCHIVES

According to Melanesian natives who preferred the position of the man kneeling between the woman's outspread legs, the missionary position only resulted in the man pressing downward, making the woman unable to respond.

HISTORICAL AND HYSTERICAL FACTS | The term "blue balls" is at least four centuries old and first appeared in England as "blue bollocks."

Though myths may be based on certain nuggets of truth or fact, they often evolve into overgeneralizations and partial truths. Obviously, this information can quickly become misleading, if not dangerous. For instance, when it was first discovered that some women were able to be multiorgasmic, this information was immediately downloaded and disseminated into the larger cultural arena as not only fact but a mandate that insisted, *If you are a real woman, you have to learn to be multiorgasmic*. Instead of presenting this information as an opportunity to explore more pleasure, the media treated it as a tool to pressure women and their partners.

Another example is the overemphasis of certain sexual discoveries. First it was the discovery of the G-spot when every magazine was telling its readers that the best orgasm came from G-spot stimulation. Well, this is all fine and good for those who experience G-spot orgasms; however, for those women who are unable to become excited by stimulation of the G-spot, all this media pressure simply makes them feel badly about themselves. Women report that such pressure makes them feel their bodies aren't okay. We all know women have already received more than their fair share of negative body images. Why add to a false sense of inadequacy with pressure on how you *should* orgasm? I agree with Dr. Bernie Zilbergeld who believes that a woman should not be tied to trying to find her G-spot. If she does or her partner does, then great. If not, there are plenty of other areas of her body to explore.

HISTORICAL AND HYSTERICAL FACTS	The know-it-alls of ancient times actually believed that every time you had an ejaculation, you lost a small amount of your brain. They called semen cerebri stillicidium, which roughly translates as "distillate of brain."

The same information backlash can negatively impact men. When a man hears that he should learn to be multiorgasmic in order to satisfy his woman, it can again trigger his performance anxiety. Sure, some men may be able to learn this technique (which essentially involves a very well-trained PC muscle that helps him refrain from ejaculating), but it is certainly not a skill required for being a wonderful, satisfying lover.

HISTORICAL AND HYSTERICAL FACTS	Elephants are only able to have erections during mating season, and they have motile penises, meaning their organs can move by themselves. This is a good thing, as they weigh a ton!

Any sexual myth does a disservice to the people who hear it by further eroding women's and men's sexual confidence, which is the key to letting go of inhibitions and exploring sexual pleasure. This is true in all areas of life: the more confidence you have, the more freedom you will experience to try new things, be it driving a car, investing in a new company, or pleasing your lover. There seems to be a direct correlation between someone's personal confidence about their sexuality and their ability to enjoy sex. Above all, I think it's important for women and men to honor and respect their own experience of sex. If something feels right and good, then do it. If something feels false, misleading, or forced, then acknowledge your feelings and back off. You are in charge; you are the ultimate authority.

Getting Beyond the Sin / Pleasure Tango

Myths also reinforce the cultural or personal barriers that prevent women and men from fulfilling their sexual potential.

Many of these myths are historical in nature and often have been tied to limiting our access or ability to feel pleasure. In his study of the history of sexuality, Dr. Mitchell Tepper, founder of sexualhealth.com, points out that the cultural or religious beliefs that said sex was bad, pleasure was a sin, and that an orgasm might as well damn you and send you straight to hell have existed throughout history. These attitudes began with the Greeks, were adopted and further developed by the Roman Catholic Church, and then were transformed and assumed by the Puritans who came to America and very much influenced our national cultural attitudes toward sex.

Take for example the sexual impulse over which Adam and Eve had no control, which was referred to as concupiscence or lust by Saint Augustine. By naming it such, lust converted procreation into something shameful, which then led to the belief that Christians should have sex without passion and only for the purpose of procreation. This dictum essentially made it sinful to find enjoyment in sex. As Dr. Tepper points out, "Americans, whether or not they are Christians, are heirs to this tradition, and understanding this background might help us to come to terms with our own ambiguous feelings about sex."

SECRET FROM LOU'S ARCHIVES

Saint Augustine felt that woman was man's greatest obstacle to salvation. This, of course, is the same man who prayed, "God, please make me chaste—but not yet."

It has only been since modern psychology started developing at the turn of the twentieth century that sexual attitudes began to shift from a sex-as-sin attitude and women and men began to think about sex in a more open way. In this country, however, it wasn't really until the women's movement that both women and men realized that sex was actually for enjoyment and that it was good for you!

<table>
<tr><td>HISTORICAL AND HYSTERICAL FACTS</td><td>Back in the Middle Ages, straight pubic hair was a sign of too much masturbation, which presumably accounts for the wide popularity of miniature pubic hair curlers at the time.</td></tr>
</table>

There have been many ways the premise that sex is a sin has affected the way we think about sex, specifically orgasms. One consequence is that in trying to control our urges, we cut off our natural sexual spontaneity. How can we feel lust and sexual pleasure if we are afraid—in some unconscious way—to let go? Without the permission to play and enjoy, you automatically cut off access to the different levels or degrees or sexual pleasure.

Read Between the Lines

I'd like to give you a little information that has contributed to the fuzziness of the information that's out there about sex. Relative to women's orgasms, there have been regular bouts of controversy within the professional fields. According to such early scientists as the psychoanalyst Sigmund Freud, orgasms resulting from stimulation of the clitoris were in some way less "mature" than orgasms originating in the vagina. Later, the research conducted by Masters and Johnson indicated that all female orgasms resulted from clitoral stimulation and refuted Freud's belief in the vaginal orgasm. Then information started to come out about the G-spot and it became clear that there is at least one area in the vagina where an orgasm can be triggered. Also, the original Masters and Johnson research did not acknowledge the existence of female ejaculation. When validation of female ejaculation first hit the airwaves and magazine stands, it spread like wildfire.

I am all for disseminating the latest sex research to mainstream publications, but I am very wary of the information being presented incompletely. Again, the idea that *all* women ejaculate during sex still holds a lot of sway, is often referred to in mainstream publications, and is often cited by doctors. However, much of this research is now considered outdated by doctors and experts, and yet, as you have seen above, there are inaccuracies that continue to exist from incomplete or outdated research.

Other examples of inaccurate reporting include Masters and Johnson's report that there is only one reflex pathway in sexual response. They maintain that since the clitoris is the major source of sensory input in women, the pudendal nerve serves as the "orgasmic platform." However, other researchers, including Dr. Beverly Whipple, have demonstrated that there are at least two nerve pathways leading women to orgasm. These include those nerves tied to the G-spot, the vagina, and the urethra.

All these researchers have made important contributions to our knowledge and understanding of sex and orgasms. However, it's important to be careful of what is reported in a sensational or incomplete manner. Read between the lines and let your own experience be your best guide.

<table>
<tr><td>

HISTORICAL AND HYSTERICAL FACTS

</td><td>

"Victoria Woodhull, prostitute, spiritualist, Wall Street broker, publisher of a national newspaper, ran for President of the United States against Ulysses S. Grant and Horace Greeley in 1872," notes Irving Wallace. "Her platform supported free love, short skirts, abolition of the death penalty, vegetarianism, excess-profit taxes, birth control, better public housing, easier divorce laws, world government, and female orgasm." Truly a woman ahead of her time.

</td></tr>
</table>

The Not-So-Subtle Power of the Media

In contemporary times, these myths continue to have power, and sometimes in dangerous ways. Essentially, many articles put pressure on women and men to perform sexually in bed and look a certain way (i.e., for women, tall, thin, and sexy; for men, muscle-bound, tall, and athletic). Neither women nor men can live up to these standards. Furthermore, by not being able to duplicate the false ideals, they feel they have failed, and end up feeling badly about themselves.

As I have mentioned before, the most oft-asked question by *Cosmo* readers is how to have an orgasm during intercourse. These young women are feeling pressured by their male partners, who are often older or more experienced, to have an orgasm in a way and manner that doesn't typically work well for women. That is, a vaginal orgasm when the man is on top during intercourse. This difficulty is further increased in this position by the man's thrusting, which creates a motion against her clitoris that doesn't work for most women. Talk about a no-win situation! The men are trying to pleasure their partners based on information they learned from adult films, and chances are good that this is bad or inaccurate information. They may also be trying to satisfy their own sexual agenda of "giving her an orgasm." This just creates performance pressure for both women and men—which further erodes the ability to access the most pleasure possible.

Who Determines What's Sexy?

Another negative aspect of the power of the media is their tendency to offer prescriptions or definitions for what is sexy. This is dangerous because if we are inundated with images or advice on how to look or act sexy, we may begin to question ourselves. If the images or advice are different from how we naturally dress or act, then we might end up feeling insecure, inadequate, or unattractive. My policy has always been if you feel sexy, you are sexy.

In my sexuality seminars, the women and men who were most confident about their sexiness-factor were those people who were at home in their own bodies. There wasn't a single look for women or for men. The range of women included Rubenesque women, short women, tall women—in every possible combination of characteristics, from curvy to boyish to angular to lean and lithe. The women who felt sexy shared an attitude about how they felt about themselves. Rather than putting on an act of bravado, "I am so hot, baby," these women seemed quietly comfortable in their own skins. Don't we all know someone who is not outwardly a "beauty" but who has always attracted men? We know intuitively that it's something about what *she knows*. And what she knows is this: She is attractive, she is sexy, she is desirable.

The same goes for men. The outwardly gorgeous guy is not necessarily the most sexy. Rather, the sexiest man alive usually is the one who sincerely likes women, wants to please women, and loves paying attention to women. Why might a woman go for a funny man? Because usually that humor is a conscious effort to amuse and delight her.

HISTORICAL AND HYSTERICAL FACTS | Among some Caribbean peoples, the husband and wife did not have intercourse at night. This was because it was believed if a child were created at night, it would surely be born blind.

Sexiness is not about looks as much as it is about knowing yourself sexually and feeling comfortable and confident in your desire to be sexual. Letting your partner know how he or she excites or attracts you is always a good idea. This kind of feedback is not about an empty gesture; it's about being honest with yourself and your partner and letting the other know what you like and what turns you on.

Our Notions of Pleasure

Before we look at exactly how to increase the number of ways you can learn to orgasm and increase the degree of pleasure you experience while doing so, I agree with Dr. Mitch Tepper that it's important to consider the nature (and notion) of pleasure itself. It's my experience that if you have a narrow view of pleasure, one restricted by either attitude or experience, then you will necessarily limit the degree to which you can feel pleasure. That said, the more open you are to pleasure—in all its forms—the more free you are to discover or deepen pleasure, especially in the sexual realm. So what is pleasure?

In his provocative discussion of the nature and notion of pleasure, Dr. Tepper cites *The Oxford English Dictionary*'s definition of pleasure as "the condition of consciousness or sensation induced by the environment or anticipation of what is felt or viewed as good or desirable; enjoyment, delight, gratification. The opposite of pain." One sexologist places pleasure in four specific categories: physiopleasure (based in the body), sociopleasure (experienced with other people), psychopleasure (emotional pleasure experienced from initiating or doing something—anything—for yourself), and ideopleasure (pleasure received from experiencing or creating something based on a theoretical idea, such as writing a book, making a movie, creating music, or constructing a building).

This use of categories suggests that we experience pleasure on different levels, which is also true of sexual pleasure. However, sexual pleasure is mostly thought of as something experienced solely in the body. In the past twenty or so years, the idea that sexual pleasure was restricted to the body began to be questioned. Specifically, in 1974, Masters and Johnson presented their findings that sexual pleasure involved the brain as much as the body, calling sexual pleasure psychophysiological and for the first time in scientific circles pointing out that sexual pleasure is experienced both in the body and in the brain. Now this may seem like common sense to most of us, but put yourself in your grandparents' generation and imagine what it would feel like to think it was either wrong or unnatural to get sexually excited in your head?!

The Masters and Johnson discovery was important because if you understand that sex happens both in the mind and the body, then you realize why negative or restrictive attitudes toward sex, absorbed from religion or basic cultural attitudes, can have such an enormous impact on us as people. If you believe that sex is dirty, that orgasms (and sexual pleasure in general) are unnecessary and an indication of a less than good character, then you will take that attitude into the bedroom with you. Having trouble letting go to feel pleasure when your husband stimulates your clitoris? Perhaps that's because you hear someone's voice insisting that you should not enjoy such stimulation.

These attitudes are both prevalent and buried deep in our culture, and while many of us consciously include ourselves in the group of the sexually liberated, it's often surprising how entrenched certain voices may be in our heads, preventing us from truly enjoying ourselves. As we will see in chapter 4, sex (and orgasms in particular) is very much a mental game. And the first step you need to take is knowing how you think and feel about sex. But one thing is for certain. As Dr. Tepper says, sexual pleasure is as unique to each person as his or her history, past learning, attitudes, and beliefs.

Why Goal-Oriented Sex Backfires

By thinking of sex as a goal-oriented event, with orgasm as the chief end, you automatically and immediately limit your ability to feel pleasure along the way. As Dr. Beverly Whipple notes in her important recent article "Beyond the G-Spot: Recent Research on Female Sexuality," there are two commonly held views of sexual activity. The more common view is goal-directed, which, she says, is "analogous to climbing the stairs." "The first step is touch, the next step is kissing, the next steps are caressing, then vagina/penis contact, which leads to intercourse and the top step of orgasm. One or both partners have a goal in mind and that goal is orgasm." According to Dr. Whipple, this goal-oriented approach to sex and, by extension, orgasm is flawed and naturally limiting to most women and men, and especially to couples.

The other view of sexuality is "pleasure-directed, . . . which can be conceptualized as a circle—with each expression on the perimeter of the circle considered an end in itself. Whether the experience is kissing or oral sex, holding, etc., each is . . . satisfying to the couple. There is no need for any particular form of expression to lead to anything else."

Dr. Whipple further points out the danger of goal-oriented sex in general: "If one person in a couple is goal oriented (typically male) and the other person is pleasure directed (typically but not always the female), problems may occur if the goals are not achieved or if the person does not communicate the goals to the partner."

Do you or your partner think of sex in this linear way? Can you see how such an attitude might prevent you from meandering along the avenue of pleasures? As universal as sex is, it is also very individualistic particularly when it comes to orgasms. Researchers Hartman, Fithian, and Campbell coined the phrase "orgasmic fingerprinting," to stress the uniqueness of each woman's orgasm. I believe in this uniqueness wholeheartedly and agree with Dr. Beverly Whipple in her strong belief that we all should have our individual, idiosyncratic sexual responses validated.

Just as we are unique human beings, so we are unique sexual creatures. Trust yourself, and your own experience—especially when it comes to sex and orgasms. In the next chapter we look more closely at the body and what is happening within it during an orgasmic response. So keep in mind as you begin to observe the body in its sexual splendor that there is no right or wrong way to enjoy pleasure or achieve an orgasm.

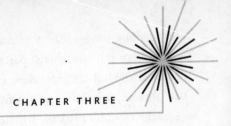

CHAPTER THREE

The Physical Side of Orgasms

The Body's Responses

Body Boldness

Most of the time, when we think about sex, specifically about orgasms, we imagine it as an activity or expression of the body. From a purely physical point of view, the body is the vehicle through which we experience pleasure.

Nowhere is the importance of knowing and being comfortable with your body more crucial than with your sexuality. And yet, in my experience, many women and men don't really know what's happening with their bodies sexually. This is in part the case because sex is a private and intimate matter, and it's rare that we feel completely free and open about discussing this area of our lives. But I also think that the lack of knowledge or familiarity with our sexual bodies is also a result of the conflicting messages and seemingly contradictory information we receive about sex. Without accurate information we are fated to remain in information limbo, not sure which way to turn to answer our questions or share our experiences.

Do you have a sense when your body is not responding sexually the way you want? Sometimes we know it's because of a recent cold or flu or feeling tired or overstressed at work. Sometimes it's a result of a recent operation or other health condition. If our body isn't working, or we are unsure of how it works sexually, then we are often cut off from fully accessing our sexual pleasure. Now, if that were the case with you or your partner, wouldn't you want to do something about it? Knowing how the body is supposed to work sexually will at the very least give you a sense of what's happening and why. And if some part of you begins to respond slowly or not at all, then you will be more aware and take the steps to ask a professional.

SECRET FROM LOU'S ARCHIVES

Dr. Herbert Otto points out that most sexologists have concluded that sex is largely a learned response. Not only are most of our sexual behavior and response patterns learned, but the orgasm as well as the possibilities of this event are also learned. The implication is that what is learned is furnished by the society in which we grew up. The question then has to be asked: "What is the content of the learning about sex which defines the parameters of a person's sexual potential?"

The Phases—Twain the Two Will Meet

In their pioneering work *Human Sexual Response*, Masters and Johnson described the physiological changes that men and women go through during sex in terms of a sexual response cycle. They arbitrarily divided this cycle into four phases:

1. Excitement or arousal
2. Plateau
3. Orgasm
4. Resolution

For the past twenty-five years, this part of their work has been widely popularized and accepted. However, many men's and women's sexual responses don't fit neatly into the Masters and Johnson paradigm. As Bernie Zilbergeld, Ph.D., points out in his groundbreaking book *The New Male Sexuality*, Alfred Kinsey is more on target: "There is nothing more characteristic of sexual response than the fact that it is not the same in any two individuals." In other words, there is no right

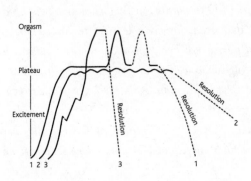

THE FEMALE SEXUAL RESPONSE CYCLE
Three representative variations of female sexual response. Pattern 1 shows multiple orgasms; pattern 2 shows arousal that reaches the plateau level without going on to orgasm (note that resolution occurs very slowly); and pattern 3 shows several brief drops in the excitement phase followed by an even more rapid resolution phase. Also note that, unlike in males, there is no refractory period in the female sexual response cycle.

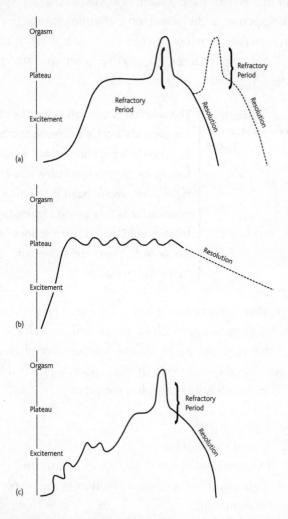

THE MALE SEXUAL RESPONSE CYCLE

(a) The most typical pattern of male sexual response. The dotted line shows one possible variation: a second orgasm and ejaculation after the refractory period is over. **(b)** Male sexual response in a situation of prolonged arousal at the plateau level not going on to orgasm and ejaculation. Note that there is no refractory period in this instance, and resolution occurs considerably more slowly. **(c)** Male sexual response pattern showing erratic initial arousal and a relatively brief plateau prior to orgasm.

or normal way to have a sexual experience. Your or your partner's response is the result of a complex interaction among many variables, including your age, your physical and emotional state, how turned on you are, what your partner does, and how you feel about him or her.

Another important sexologist, Dr. Lasse Hessel, presents a slightly different approach to men's and women's sexual cycles. He divides the act of making love into five phases, which he says, "is, of course, very theoretical division, as the phases merge into each other, one after the other."

1. Foreplay
2. Sexual stimulation
3. Dilation (expansion of the upper part of the vagina in the woman and erection in the man)
4. Orgasm/climax
5. Relaxation

For Dr. Hessel, the distinction between foreplay and sexual stimulation is important because it underscores that becoming aroused with your partner is both a mental and physical activity. In foreplay, Hessel maintains, couples excite and prepare each other for having sex, using their own rituals or sexual code. This happens at a more mental and emotional level. In the next phase, couples sexually stimulate each other by touching, kissing, or any other way that gets their bodies sexually aroused so that blood flow to the genitals increases. In the third phase, blood flow increases to such a degree that genitals are fully engorged with blood—for the woman, her vagina and clitoris are enlarged and aroused; for the man, his penis has become erect and his scrotum swells or lifts.

The fourth phase is orgasm and the fifth and last phase is relaxation, similar to what Masters and Johnson call resolution. My point here is to show you that even though there are some universal patterns that indicate sexual excitement and the steps leading toward orgasm, many experts distinguish the phases differently, emphasizing their own particular point of view.

I think what's important is becoming familiar with the general sexual flow so that you are comfortable with all aspects of your sexual experience. A question for all of us is, how can we help our partner reach an orgasm if we've rushed through foreplay? Gentlemen, this is especially true if you haven't given a woman time to warm up. And ladies, do you really want to take away your man's pleasure by pushing him toward climax when, at that time, he seems to be enjoying being touched, caressed, and fondled by you?

Dr. Hessel points out that "exciting and fulfilling lovemaking takes more than just knowing how to treat your partner physically in order for you both to achieve orgasm." Foreplay is at least as important and pleasurable as intercourse, and it is essential to remember that the same things are not necessarily as sexually stimulating for the woman as they are for the man. Normally, the woman takes much longer to reach the same level of arousal as the man. The considerate and caring man will have to restrain his own needs so that the woman can gradually build up her level of sexual arousal.

SECRET FROM LOU'S ARCHIVES

Any sexual experience has the right to be validated as good, great, or okay. I agree strongly with Dr. Beverly Whipple, who said, "Our objective has been to validate women's accounts of their sexual experiences, not create new goals."

While many of us may recognize these differing definitions, my point is to at once offer you a general framework from which to become aware of your own sexual cycles and bring to light the shades of gray when it comes to pinpointing an exact cycle that matches all women and all men. Matching, it appears from the research, is a rarity. Use the information as a way to become more aware of and therefore in tune with your own orgasmic potential.

Men's Sexual Cycle

The main physical changes that occur in men's bodies during a sexual experience are the result of vasocongestion, or the accumulation of blood in various parts of the body. Muscle tension increases and other changes, such as increased respiration and pulse rate, also occur. With orgasm, the muscular tension is released or discharged and blood flow resumes its normal or resting rate.

Arousal

For both men and women, a sexual response begins when you receive some kind of sexual stimulation: a touch, smell, sight, thought, fantasy, or anything that has erotic meaning for you—and given the range of ideas floating around in our heads, just about anything might have erotic meaning for us. As a result of this stimulation, the brain triggers an increased volume of blood to be pumped into various parts of your body, increasing most obviously the size of the genitals. As a result of this increase in blood flow, the genitals become darker and even more sensitive to stimulation. It goes without saying that Mother Nature really knew what she was doing here.

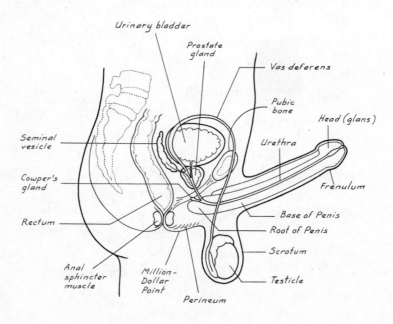

Male Genitalia

Male Physical Response

EXCITEMENT

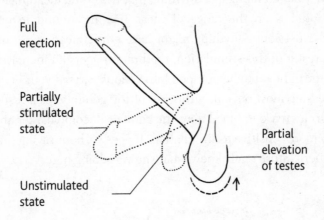

Full erection

Partially stimulated state

Partial elevation of testes

Unstimulated state

PLATEAU

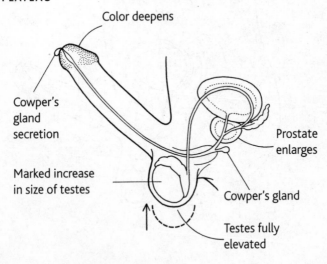

Color deepens

Cowper's gland secretion

Prostate enlarges

Marked increase in size of testes

Cowper's gland

Testes fully elevated

ORGASM

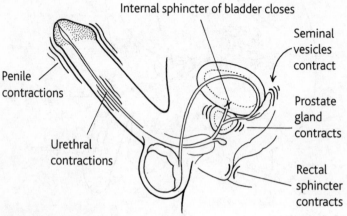

Internal sphincter of bladder closes

Seminal vesicles contract

Penile contractions

Prostate gland contracts

Urethral contractions

Rectal sphincter contracts

Contractions force the seminal fluid through the urethra

RESOLUTION

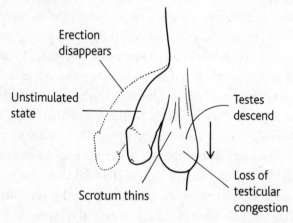

Erection disappears

Unstimulated state

Testes descend

Loss of testicular congestion

Scrotum thins

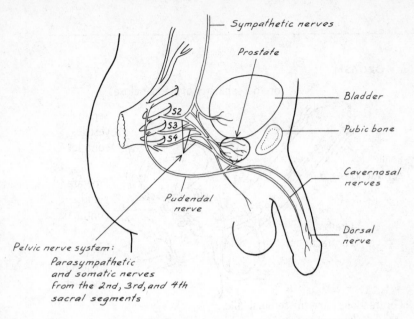

Male Sexual Nerve Arrangement

Your penis, your lips, earlobes, and nipples all receive more blood flow, making them more alert and receptive to touch or stimulation. Have you ever noticed that when your partner touches your arm while you are kissing or beginning to make love that you suddenly feel the hair stand up on end, as if suddenly your entire arm has become an erogenous zone?! Other areas such as your breasts (this is true for men and women) also become aroused, and change form. The scrotal sac, for instance, thickens and contracts, while the testes increase in size with the engorgement of blood. The testes are also pulled up within the sac until they press against the wall of the pelvis. It is the thin layer of muscle within the scrotum called the cremasteric muscle that does this. This elevation of the testes anticipates ejaculation and is necessary for it to occur.

Erection

A penis's erection is really a study in fluid hydraulics. With each wave of stimulation, the brain signals there to be a commensurate flow of blood into the three main spongy tissue chambers of the penis. When these are filled (fully engorged), an erection occurs. A penis also has a regular cycle of nocturnal erections, which explains why men will often wake with an erection. This doesn't necessarily mean they were having wild sex dreams; it's simply nature's way of maintaining good, healthy penis tissue.

When a large amount of blood flows into the penis (without flowing out again) the penis becomes erect. Full erection may or may not occur early in an experience. In many young men, erection is almost instantaneous; they get hard as soon as they get any stimulation. With increasing age, however, it usually takes longer to get hard, and even direct stimulation of the penis may not be enough to make a man erect. As men age, their sexual reactions become more in line with women, especially in terms of timing. I've been told this is nature's way of leveling the playing field. Older men are more easily distracted and require more direct stimulation to become and stay erect. (We'll discuss medical issues such as impotence and premature ejaculation later, in chapter 7.)

Many factors can affect a man's ability to become erect. Anxiety, stress, or simply becoming distracted. As one man put it, "When I am stressed about work, it is like my equipment doesn't work." As the experts say, anxiety can cause loss of both erection and ejaculation. Another man said this: "When I am angry, I can still get up to do the job. But I'm definitely not as there mentally." Strong emotion is a natural distraction to sex, especially if the emotion is caused by something outside the sexual or romantic moment.

Ejaculation

Ejaculation is a spinal reflex that releases the built-up muscular tension and reverses blood flow in the body, draining it away from the penis and other engorged areas. Two distinct steps are involved in ejaculation: First, the prostate, seminal vesicles, and vas deferens contract, pouring their contents into the urethra. The sperm mix with the secretions of the seminal vesicles and the prostate to form the ejaculate.

The contractions are the beginning of the ejaculation. This is when men say they feel they're about to come. Masters and Johnson call this point of the phase "ejaculatory inevitability," because once the contractions begin, the process usually happens involuntarily.

During the second step of the ejaculatory process, the fluid is propelled through the urethra by contractions of the pelvic muscles (the PC muscles). The semen may spurt several inches or even feet beyond the tip of the penis, or it may simply seep or trickle out. Of course, I've noted in my research that many men have claimed great distances, high jumpers I like to call them. The amount and force of ejaculate expelled are determined by a number of factors, including age, general health, and the length of time since the last ejaculation. Anecdotally, there seems to be correlation between how young you are and the greater distance your semen will travel. Also, if you haven't come in a long time, you will also tend to have more semen built up, ready to be released.

Although ejaculation occurs in and through the penis, it is in fact a "total-body response," according to Dr. Bernie Zilbergeld. Respiration, blood pressure, and heartbeat increase as a man approaches ejaculation, usually peaking at the moment of "propulsion." But many men have reported (to me), "At that moment, I don't know anything else in the world except that sensation." Another male seminar attendee said, "Sometimes I think it is going to be a great one, and then it just sort of pffts out—there just isn't enough flow. Those are rather disappointing." While I understand the man's disappointment, it's important for him to know that this is perfectly natural and certainly not a reflection of his manhood or sexual prowess.

Resolution

After ejaculation, a man's body starts to return to its equilibrium, or prearoused state. For most men, this move (what Masters and Johnson refer to as the shift from orgasm to resolution) happens very quickly, hence the clichéd image of men falling into a deep slumber once they come. One man explained the feeling this way: "After I have an orgasm, every ounce of stress in my body is gone for the next twenty-five minutes."

SECRET FROM LOU'S ARCHIVES

Oftentimes women will ask why men fall asleep right after sex. From what I can deduce, put someone in a darkened room at the end of the day, give them a tremendous physical sensation that results in complete relaxation, and sleep is likely. Think of how you feel after a massage: Do you really want to go out dancing?!

What's really happening in the body is that after ejaculation, the blood flows out of the penis, which then returns to a flaccid (nonerect) state. Blood pressure, pulse, and breathing rates also return to normal. The scrotum and testes lose their engorgement and become smaller in size and return to their normal position. The reason many men feel as if they could sleep is because of a deep state of relaxation—they've just built up and then released tremendous muscle tension, giving them an overall body relaxation. Think of how you feel after a workout: Once your body is moved, manipulated, and stretched, don't you then feel an all-around sense of relaxation?

Women's Sexual Cycle

Like a man's cycle, a woman goes through the four basic phases from arousal through climax to resolution. However, as we saw earlier in this chapter, this cycle is rarely in sync with a man's.

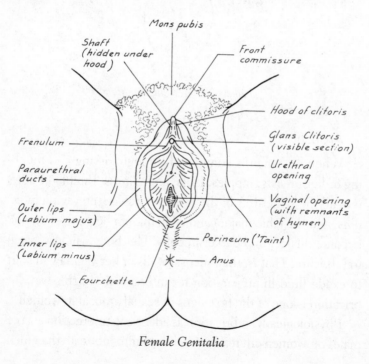

Female Genitalia

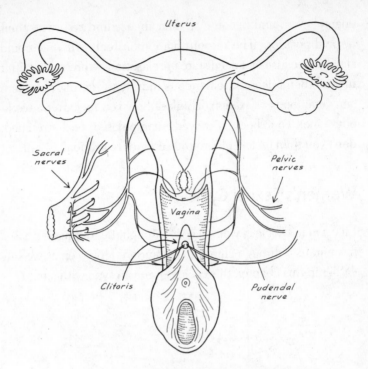

Female Nerve Arrangement

Arousal

When a woman is stimulated through kissing and touching of her breasts, nipples, labia, and clitoris, the blood flows into all the structures of the woman's pelvis, the vagina moistens, and the labia majora and labia minora begin to swell and become duskier and darker in color. Her body will also begin to lubricate. That is, the mucosal walls of her vagina will start to exude fluid in preparation for intercourse. In this way, lubrication is one of the first signs of sexual arousal in women.

Physiologically, lubrication is identical to erection in the male, yet women often take much longer to lubricate than men take to get an erection. Women's bodies will naturally respond as they were designed to during arousal, but often men will seem to be way ahead of them—a man may be erect and ready to go while the woman is still getting warmed up. Although some women will begin to lubricate within thirty seconds of being stimulated—either mentally or physically—not all women do. Some may take several minutes or not lubricate at all. So please don't use this as the only criteria for assessing whether you are ready or not.

<table>
<tr><td>HISTORICAL AND HYSTERICAL FACTS</td><td>According to Drs. Joel Block and Susan Crain Bakos, "women's increased ease with their bodies and confidence in lovemaking continues to grow after their thirties. And a woman's orgasmic capacity including the ability to have multiple orgasms is undiminished by age." However, a "man cannot be truly said to peak until he has become a good, even a great, lover with ejaculatory control and the ability to please his partner in different ways and that is unlikely to happen at nineteen."</td></tr>
</table>

Sometimes women, no matter how aroused they may be in their heads, may still be dry and unable to lubricate. This can be caused by a range of things, including medications, such as antihistamines, which dry out body tissues, to how hydrated she is. If she has drunk any alcohol during the evening, she may be slightly dehydrated, which will directly affect her ability to lubricate. This reaction is also true of smoking or by a

Female Physical Response

EXCITEMENT

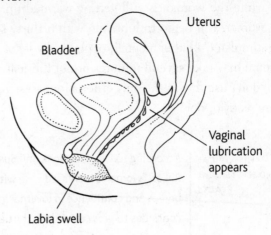

Uterus

Bladder

Vaginal lubrication appears

Labia swell

PLATEAU

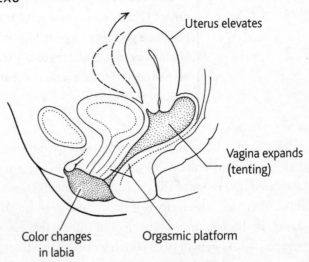

Uterus elevates

Vagina expands (tenting)

Color changes in labia

Orgasmic platform

ORGASM

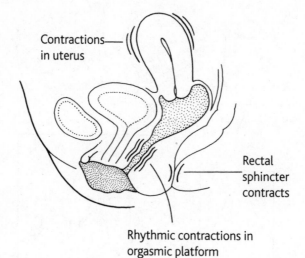

Contractions in uterus

Rectal sphincter contracts

Rhythmic contractions in orgasmic platform

RESOLUTION

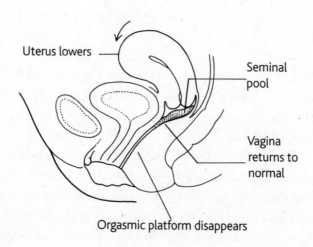

Uterus lowers

Seminal pool

Vagina returns to normal

Orgasmic platform disappears

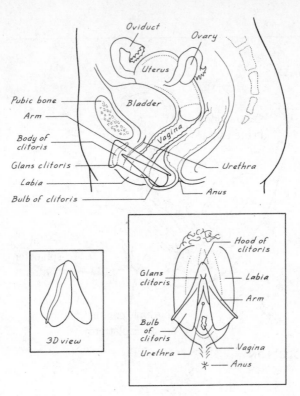

The Clitoris

lack of the hormone estrogen, which is essential for lubrication. In chapter 8, I offer a number of wonderful lubricants that can be used for intercourse, manual stimulation, oral sex, and with toys.

The second stage of arousal for women is when the vagina elongates and the uterus has moved up and out of the way, ballooning in the upper third to make room for the penis. You may be unaware, as most women are, of this internal change in your vagina, especially after your partner has entered you, when you become even more stimulated.

Orgasm

From the strictly physiologic point of view, a woman's orgasm is marked by the muscles of the upper third of the vagina and the uterus beginning to contract. But a lot more is going on; this is what is happening in her body as she reaches climax:

1. Muscles tense and heart rate and blood pressure increase.
2. Nipples become erect.
3. The blood-engorged clitoris becomes erect and pulls under the clitoral hood.
4. The labia majora and labia minora enlarge and lubrication increases.
5. The vagina continues to expand and lengthen and breasts engorge slightly.
6. The clitoris shortens; the color of the labia deepens.
7. Muscles, including the anal sphincter, continue to tense and then contract, sometimes spasming.
8. Orgasm or release occurs (contractions increase to every .8 seconds).

Orgasms can be big or small, short or long, and as you will see in chapter 5, women can experience up to ten different types of orgasms! While I will go into this subject in much greater length in chapter 7, I do want to stress that some women who have never experienced an orgasm feel that their lack of response is related to never having the safety of a secure sexual relationship in which to explore how they like to be touched. Still other women feel they are anorgasmic (the inability to orgasm) because they suffered some kind of emotional or sexual abuse. I'm sure that as our scientific insight into orgasm progresses, we will begin to understand more fully why some women are unable to have an orgasm. But please keep in mind that although orgasms follow a very concrete physiological course, they also possess an enormous emotional and psychological component. If you are a woman who has not yet experienced an orgasm, do not give up hope. An orgasm is not only possible, it's probable.

HISTORICAL AND HYSTERICAL FACTS	The Dutch physician Regnier de Graaf first mentioned female ejaculation in 1672.

Female Ejaculation

Recent research has documented female ejaculation and actually analyzed the fluid that is emitted. The liquid was found to contain a chemical, acid phosphatase, which is only found in one other gland, the male prostate. Francisco Cabello Santa Maria, a Spanish sex researcher, showed that the fluid ejaculated by women contained PSA, prostatic specific antigen. This finding came from a study in which women were masturbating, therefore eliminating the possibility that a man's fluid may somehow have appeared on the scene. This finding also implies the existence of glands along the urethra, the channel from the bladder, which produce the fluid for female ejaculation. As Dr. Lana Holstein points out in her book, *How to Have Magnificent Sex*, many women have found that stimulation of the clitoris produces this release. Other women feel the urge to bear down as they feel this swelling from increased stimulation in the vagina, which can also produce the ejaculation. Women describe the sensation of ejaculation as a pushing down and an overall bodily releasing sensation. And some women say that this state is a much more intense and satisfying orgasm.

As I indicated in chapter 2, a woman may be made to think that she has urinated because neither the man nor the woman know at the time what is happening. Again, Dr. Holstein says that "most women who ejaculate explain that it occurs when they feel safe and free with a partner and happens only when they are certain that it will not be viewed with alarm." Dr. Holstein suggests that if you know you may ejaculate, try putting a towel under your hips. Then, if you ejaculate—or if you want to use massage oil or a vaginal lubricant—you won't have to be thinking about the laundry.

Resolution

The last stage of the sexual response is when all of the changes you experienced from increased heart rate to pelvic blood flow return to normal. Women often feel a surge of energy following orgasm. In fact some women have said they feel more awake: "I am more in tune with everything. Unfortunately, this tends to happen at night. But otherwise, what a jolt!" Another woman said this: "Sometimes when we make love I feel so connected to my husband that it is like I want to be inside his skin. The feeling of coming and being that close to him is electric."

How Should We Define an Orgasm?

As Dr. Mitch Tepper points out, Masters and Johnson describe orgasm as strictly mechanical (i.e., muscular) and hydraulic (i.e., related to blood flow). This definition neatly leaves out any psychological or emotional dimension or aspect contributing to orgasm. This is important because of the prevalent and pervasive effect of Masters and Johnson's research on other thinkers. As I said earlier in chapter 2, if we think of orgasm in such a limited way, won't we also experience orgasms in a limited way?

Those researchers who have a psychological point of view see orgasm as "peaking of sexual pleasure with a release of sexual tension and rhythmic contraction of the perineal muscles and reproductive organs." I find both these definitions so pinpoint specific that they limit the possible range of orgasms women and men can experience. I would rather adopt a definition that includes a range of points, so that both the psychological (mental and emotional) aspects of orgasm as well as its physiological connections are emphasized. This is vital to being able to tap into your individual sexual pleasure—in whatever form that exists. Blending the two points of view encourages all women and men to experience and take pleasure in whatever they wish.

Orgasms clearly happen in the body and through the body. However, for all their physiological reality, they also have a very real mental (both psychological and emotional) dimension. Want to know why the brain has often been called the body's most important sex organ? Just wait and see.

CHAPTER FOUR

Clearing Your Head

The Mental Side of Orgasms

Turning the Tables on Performance Anxiety

We've all heard that the power or control of an orgasm is tied to our brains, which makes all kinds of sense, as our brain is our most powerful sex organ. We hear, too, that many women and men are stressed about orgasms and can experience a tremendous amount of performance anxiety when it comes to giving or having an orgasm. In my seminars I hear time and again how afraid women and men are to even try, for fear of being disappointed themselves or disappointing their lovers. I say throw away all of this negative energy around orgasms out the window. We've become a nation of people sexually trying to keep up with the Joneses, who live down the street and are having amazing sex every night of the week, with awesome transportive orgasms. Well, might I suggest we know it doesn't serve us to try to keep up with the Joneses relative to material possessions, so let's not do the same relative to sex.

Although I believe that there can be a serious side to orgasms, sometimes deep and life altering, I think that if we focus too much on anticipating, controlling, or examining our orgasms, then we not only put enormous pressure on ourselves to have one, we also take the fun and enjoyment out of it! For heaven's sake, there is plenty out there telling us what we are supposed to be experiencing and the majority is marketing hype. I mean really, how many people look like the swooning "oh baby" couples that are used to market videos to us? It is difficult when we have the ever-so-charming fear-factor style of telling us we had better do X, Y, Z or our partners will be dissatisfied and leave us.

> ### SECRET FROM LOU'S ARCHIVES
>
> *Sexual dissatisfaction isn't the thing that makes couples divorce . . . stray yes, divorce, no.*

As we saw in chapter 2, there are many misconceptions and myths about the negative aspects or limitations of sex that are still embedded in our culture and therefore our minds. Hopefully now you are more attuned to those attitudes or beliefs that you consciously or unconsciously adopted and may now feel motivated to dislodge any attitude or belief that gets in your way of fully experiencing sexual pleasure and orgasm.

The point of this chapter is to turn the negative to positive and give you the tools to better access the orgasm you want. I've tried to keep the information simple, straightforward, and fun so you can accept, enjoy, and revel in the orgasms you do have.

The Role of Communication

Speak Now or Forever Hold Thy Peace

How can you expect your partner to miraculously pleasure you the way you like to be pleasured unless you've given him or her the information? Don't you want your partner to know how to do what works for you? And don't you want to know how to do the same for your partner? We can't read our partners' minds, so why expect them to be able to do so for us? As one man from a seminar said, "I can't believe that I spent years expecting my wife to know what I wanted and how I wanted to be touched; it was like I figured if she really loved me, she would know what I liked and what I wanted." Believe me, ladies and gentlemen, in this case, love has nothing to do with it. You can't know through osmosis; you've got to communicate—either in words or through your actions. Remember show-and-tell?

> **HISTORICAL AND HYSTERICAL FACTS** | Death during orgasm is a fairly uncommon event. Factors that can contribute are alcohol ingestion, food consumption, and an extramarital partner.

The key to achieving the best orgasm possible is for you to share as much as you honestly can with your lover. First you need to know yourself, know what you like, how you prefer to be touched, caressed, kissed, or licked, and then you need to share this information with your partner. Know that sharing need not be a conversation; it can be a physical motion or action. Also, for those of us who are intimidated by what we don't know and think we should know, keep in mind that although we are all born of sexuality, none of us are born knowing how to have sex. We all have to learn. And what works for one may not work for another. So as they say, every journey begins with the first step and this may well be yours in the area of knowing yourself sexually.

Most women say that in order to share or be open verbally with their partner, they have to feel safe. A woman from one of my seminars explained why even though she was attracted to a certain man, she was still unable to open herself sexually with him. "He was charming, sophisticated, great looking, and French to boot. But I simply didn't feel safe with him. I knew he had been seeing another woman and even though he professed it was over, his actions didn't make me feel safe. I couldn't relax enough to consider even getting into bed with him. Could I imagine what he would be like? Oh yeah! But in reality it was too scary, too not okay for me."

Another married woman underscored how emotionally complicated it feels to be honest with her partner: "My husband has always been the initiator in sex and I know there are things I'd like to try, but I worry he'll feel badly if I say I want to do something. I don't want him to think that he hasn't been good enough for me and then he could also think I have done something with someone else when of course I haven't." I've heard many women and men speak of their hesitation to be direct about what they want. Afraid to hurt a partner's feelings, they sacrifice their own pleasure. But take a moment here: Don't you think if you bring up the idea of your pleasure in a "hey, let's have more fun" kind of way, he or she will be turned on rather than turned off?

You won't know until you try. Consider what one woman said: "I fell in love with my husband because he had the most open, nonjudgmental attitude that I had ever encountered. The more I got to know him, the more I realized he had this attitude in all areas of his life. What a gold mine! But what I remember best is the first time he told me, 'Whatever you want a man to do to a woman, I will do. Whatever you want to do to a man, you can do to me. Baby, if you want me to bark like a dog I'll do it—'cause I'm your man.' He said this to me over the phone—I got the shivers!"

SECRET FROM LOU'S ARCHIVES

A hallmark 1986 study involving over two hundred married women reached the following conclusion: ". . . sexual fantasies help many married women to achieve sexual arousal and/or orgasm during sexual intercourse, irrespective of their current sex life status."

Testing the Waters of Compatibility

Although I think in most relationships, especially those where trust and commitment have already been established, openness is the best policy, sometimes it's also a matter of compatibility. Many men say that they don't want to alienate their partners by asking for "too much" or say that by asking, their wives or girlfriends will feel pressure. Men are aware that they ride a thin line between wanting to ask for what they want and not offending their partners. Any man knows the woman in his life controls the access to the "prize," and he has to remove as many impediments to that access as possible. One of these impediments is his fear of upsetting her. We all have an awareness that there is a range of sexual activity and fantasy that is acceptable. One man described his situation by saying, "For me, the reason I hold back is if she rejects me one night, I'll never want to try again." Obviously there is a risk of offending or hurting someone. But if you are careful and considerate in how you suggest a certain position, toy, or fantasy, there is more chance for success or at the very least an understanding "no, not tonight, honey, but maybe some other time."

Another man expressed his dilemma this way: "I knew I would never again ask this woman to try one of my favorite things [he wanted her to use a small anal vibrator on him while she was performing oral sex]. After a year and a half, I learned in that one reaction she and I wouldn't make it. I thought she was it."

SECRET FROM LOU'S ARCHIVES

*Boredom is one of the
biggest robbers of intimacy.*

It makes total sense that revealing what you want sexually can make you feel wide open and vulnerable—this is one of the great paradoxes of wonderful, gratifying sex. To feel vulnerable is only normal; after all, it is not every day we are as we came into the world—naked—with another person exploring our body in ways we may not have. The good part about vulnerability is that it flows both ways. You can have yours and your partner can have his or hers. Yet how you both react to something can either give each of you the space you need or shut you both down.

Whether you are in a long-term relationship or a brand-spanking-new one, you both can benefit from the "sharing principle." I have witnessed in my seminars that those people who risk sharing this most intimate side of themselves are invariably rewarded by being able to create an even more trusting, passionate, and charged sexual relationship. The following is a great comment from a therapist: "Showing your vulnerability creates space for someone to see where they can move into and impact your life. If the space isn't there, they can't show up—be it emotionally, psychologically, or physically."

Fun Sex or Deep Sex?
Are You and Your Partner on the Same Page?

On the road to orgasm, I think it's important that you and your partner know where you both are coming from. If you're in a playful, let's-get-hot mood, and she is in a more relaxed, romantic mood, you might encounter a bit of tension. It only makes sense that two people are not always going to be in the same kind of mood, with the same exact expectations of how, where, or what they want to do for sex. Fortunately, Mother Nature didn't make us all alike (identical twins aside), so from the git-go, two people are not going to have exactly the same sex drives or attitudes and even identical twins, like my sister and I, have very different preferences. To further complicate this situation, the number of demands and stresses we all have to deal with on a daily basis underscores the need for couples to be up-front about where they are and what they need sexually.

The suggestions below will help you both clear your heads and at the very least give you a way of finding out what is going on with each other. At the very most, you will learn that you are both on the same page, and heading to the bedroom will never feel so enticing or exciting.

Opening the Channels

As I've been saying throughout this book, when you think of orgasms as the one and only goal of sex, you greatly limit yourself to the overall sensations of sex. Specifically, as you will see in the next two chapters, in which I describe the ten different types of orgasms women can experience and the seven different types of orgasms men can experience, there is much more to sex than your old standby.

The more you involve your entire body in sex, the more likely you will open other avenues of pleasure and sensation. One woman used this example: "There is something about how my boyfriend massages my neck that causes me to melt. He is good with his hands, but this is beyond! And if we go on to have sex, it feels bigger for me."

One man pointed out how important relaxation is to a woman when he said, "What I know about my wife is if she isn't relaxed enough, nothing is going to happen. If I start to give her a foot massage as soon as she sits down on the sofa after work, she is invariably turned on. She knows I care about her, and this works!"

Keeping It Spontaneous

In the years that I've been giving sexuality seminars to hundreds—thousands—of men and women, the number one comment I hear is how much they want the heat and spontaneity back in their relationship. Once the proverbial honeymoon is over, how can a loving, committed couple keep their sexual relationship playful, fun, and zinging with that passionate energy they knew in the early years of their courtship?

Anyone who has been together five months, five years, or forty-five years knows that both people need to work at keeping the sexual relationship new and fresh, and the biggest thing that keeps sex fresh is your attitude. Quite simply, you have to make intimacy and private time together a priority. You have to do this consciously. When you were dating, romance and getting it on was a natural priority. It was an automatic.

Later on, as time passes, and the two of you become more familiar to each other, you have to make a conscious effort, including scheduling sex.

Couples also need to consciously set aside time for intimacy. Anyone who is a parent knows all about juggling timetables and the necessity for being organized. You have to stick to some sort of a timetable to keep all the machinery of a family running. The same is true for sex. By making it part of your day or week, you not only have sex, but you and your partner will connect better, and all other aspects of your life will likely fall into place. Couples without kids need to make the same consideration: Sex is a vital priority in your relationship. As one woman, a mother of three small children, said, "That, my dear, is why my husband and I have a date every Wednesday night and why my office doubles as our secret hideaway."

The threat of boring sex can freeze people internally. Sometimes women are so focused on pleasing their partners that they lose touch with their own sexual desires. Men are just as susceptible. When a man is more concerned with pleasing his woman, he can forget to access his own pleasure. My advice is to stay in your body. Stay with your own sensation. One of the biggest turn-ons for your partner is getting you turned on and knowing you are into it.

SECRET FROM LOU'S ARCHIVES

So many men take for granted that their own pleasure will be taken care of if they just focus on pleasing the woman. But it's just as important for a man to take care of himself and explore his own pleasure avenues as it is for a woman to do so.

Don't Take It Home with You

Does this sound familiar? You've just had a long, hard day at the office. You have spent the last month or so on a project and when you present it to your boss, he shoots it down and gives you your walking papers. When you go home that evening, trying to get yourself in the mood for some tender love-making with your partner, you realize that nothing is happening down there.

Many men and women are prone or sensitive to taking outside stress (particularly when they experience any kind of failure) into the bedroom. This is as much true for women who have full, complicated careers as it is for women who are mothers who stay at home. Whether it's an ever-increasing workload or the stress of caring for children, these outside distractions can interfere with sexual desire. There's no doubt about it, work and children often get in the way of feeling up for sex.

HISTORICAL AND HYSTERICAL FACTS	Having your children sleep with you is the ultimate form of birth control.

We often rely on the age-old excuse "I'm too tired" to postpone or avoid sex. Admittedly, it is sometimes hard not to let the aggravations of the day get to you. But if you treat your sexual relationship with your partner as a sanctuary, a place that gives energy instead of takes energy, then you can overcome the excuses. Right before you say no to sex, stop and think about how good you will feel afterward. Then consider saying yes. Whether it's a place and time for you both to go a little wild, rekindle the romantic fire, or create a bubble of bliss, chances are you will feel revitalized, energized, and connected when you go there.

Getting in the Mood

Enhancing your sexual pleasure also means making sure that you and your partner are in the mood. For women, this is especially important since one of the most important elements of a woman enjoying herself sexually depends on her degree of relaxation. If a woman is not relaxed enough, chances are she won't be able to get turned on enough to really get into sex. Or she may agree to it but only "go through the motions," which will damage intimacy and her sex life over time if it occurs too frequently. As I've heard over and over again from the men in my seminars, men are completely turned on by women who are into it!

But let's not forget about you gentlemen. I've also found in my research that it's equally important on occasion for the woman to take control of getting her man in the mood. The number one turn-on for men who are in an ongoing relationship is knowing they are coming home to a peaceful place. A man will do just about anything to keep peace in the household, including vacationing with his partner's friends and giving up his two-seater for a minivan; the need for peace can go deep. A man experiences being peaceful as having more access to intimacy, which, of course, leads to sex.

The best policy for creating a peaceful environment begins with stopping the inclination to bring up the problems of the day as soon as he sets foot in the door. Let him have a peaceful place in which to arrive. In no way am I suggesting that you should not talk about what you need to, but wait until you both have decompressed. Touch each other, put your hand on the back of his neck. Connect with him. This need only take five or ten minutes, perhaps longer, but then he'll be more open to what you have to say.

So, does he respond to candlelight? Does she love a foot massage or a large tumbler of water or something stronger as she walks in the door? Do you both respond to soft music and dim lighting? Does he like you in sheer black lingerie? Does she like you freshly showered and in your bathrobe? A dinner out or a home-cooked meal? Although women have been socialized to think they are the only ones who need to be romanced, men like this same kind of attention too!

Some women have come to think they alone are gift enough and that only the men should worry about being gift bearers. Not so, ladies. Women also need to be in charge of romancing and seducing their men. I have been asked repeatedly by men in my seminars and during interviews, "How can I get her to initiate sex more often? I love it when I do it, but I want her to do it to me sometimes as well." The Greatest Gift for a man may very well be the woman initiating and letting him know she is in the mood—for him. He wants to know you want him. Show him.

Romance the Dance

Relax Her

It bears repeating that if a woman isn't relaxed—physically and mentally—then it will be nearly impossible for her to become aroused sexually. So if a man wants to have sex, wants to bring his woman to heights of pleasure, then he needs to spend the time and energy focusing on her. Granted most men find the act of pleasuring her a huge turn-on, so this advice works for both of you.

First, a man needs to be a gentleman and court her. If red jujubes are her favorite, then give them to her. Any gesture that makes her feel special and heard will likely warm her and have her be more open to sex. If she likes flowers, then bring her flowers. Maybe she likes to take a bath, or simply make an occasion out of a Friday-night dinner. Paying this kind of attention will not only make her feel special, it will also make her feel warm and generous.

SECRET FROM LOU'S ARCHIVES

Follow the fashionable tradition of sixteenth- and seventeenth-century European courts and do a little courtly dressing of your pubic hair. This is particularly effective if it is something you wouldn't normally do. Ideas? Add a line of Swarovski crystal tattoo (as discussed in chapter 8) to the top of your pubic triangle. Trim it in the shape of a heart.

Gentlemen, let your women know you are doing something especially for them. When was the last time you put air in the tires or filled the gas tank for her? In your mind, you might have the intention of wanting your wife to be safe on the road. But instead of simply thinking about it, do something. I am not saying that a woman isn't fully capable of taking care of her own safety, but rather that when a woman sees her man taking care of her, she feels safe. And safety is very close to sexiness.

Mind you, I am not promoting manipulative tricks here. I am simply underscoring certain simple ways that most women like to be treated. This kind of treatment can also take place at any level: set candles around the bedroom (or any room for that matter); if you run her a bath, add a scented oil or bath foam.

But there is a practical side to getting her in the mood. Many women set foot in the proverbial door and all they can think of is the list of things they have to do before going to bed: make dinner, do the laundry, clean the house, feed and bathe the kids, return phone calls—the list can be endless. Your task, gentlemen, is to alleviate this burden and get rid of the distractions! If your partner walks in the door and there is nothing or very little for her to do, chances are she will be much more open to being romanced and seduced.

Seduce Him

Men like to get excited. No, let me change that: Men love to get excited. They also like to be treated nicely. If you know how your man likes to be romanced, then romance him in that way. Does he love an old James Dean flick? Rent one. If you know he loves a bike mag about shovelheads, buy it.

Whatever it is, the underlying ingredient to seduction (for either sex) is thoughtfulness. Most men are completely turned on by a meal you prepare for them—whether that is an elegant feast or two tacos. If you don't have time for tearing apart your kitchen, then choose a spot and make a dinner reservation. Maybe even pick him up at work. If you don't have time to change in to a sexy number that lets him know what you have in mind, then add an accessory that will catch his eye. If you are wearing a skirt, change your hose into a pair with a seam running up the back. Trust me, he will notice. Or wear stockings that hug the tops of your thighs. During dinner, place his hand on your thigh and let him feel the slight ridge at the top of the stockings. Men are masterful at knowing what is under a woman's garment, and it never hurts to prime their imaginations.

Men fantasize through their eyes as well as their ears. Across the dinner table, tell him he has complete access to you. Let him know you were just waxed this afternoon—in his favorite style—or that you thought about him as you put on your gartered nylons.

If you've planned an encounter at home (with or without toys), why not leave a coded message on his voice mail at work early in the day. It is most unlikely he will be late.

While you undress him, tell him what you want to do to him. Most men like to hear a woman talk about sex—and if you're comfortable, you can even make it a little dirty.

Being open, honest, and tactful are the three keys to good communication. And without strong communication, your chances for having mind-blowing sex decrease. So go for the gold! Share your ideas and fantasies with your partner in a tactful and respectful manner—who knows the boundaries you might cross together. This kind of sharing also increases your sexual confidence, which is so important to feeling sexy and desirable. Once you're in the right mind-set, the rest (of sex) will begin to flow. Now, are you ready for the ten different ways a woman can orgasm?

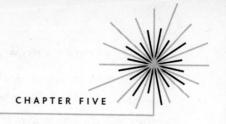

CHAPTER FIVE

The Female Orgasm

Going for the Unexpected

The Last Frontier

The female orgasm is one of the last frontiers of sexuality. In general, the average person knows less about the female orgasm—its causes, frequency, locations—than any other aspect of sex. This makes sense, because the long-term concentration of sexual research has been based on male norms. For years women have been given contradictory and inaccurate information about their orgasms by their mothers, their physicians, their partners, and anyone else who was trying to control female sexuality. Women, over time, have been convinced that orgasms were not important, that they prevented pregnancy, that they were necessary for pregnancy, that they were a sign of a "loose" woman, and finally, that they were not proper behavior.

The tides thankfully have turned. However, in more recent times, in place of myths, women have begun to feel increasing pressure to orgasm. Like men, women say they feel a certain amount of performance anxiety when it comes to frequency of orgasm and the timing of their orgasm—basically, they feel pressured to produce orgasms on demand.

HISTORICAL AND HYSTERICAL FACTS	Hippocrates apparently described the clitoris four hundred years before Christ.

I'm going to lift the lid off these misconceptions so that you will get the broadest, most comprehensive, and latest information about orgasms. This is information that will validate, empower, and enhance the orgasms you already have and possibly create new ways to experience them. This information is for you: consider it, mull it over, share it in any way, any time, any place you want to have one—or more for that matter.

Again, I am a strong believer in the policy that the more you know about any subject, distributor caps included, the more confidence you will have talking about and exploring the subject area. So the more knowledge you have about your body and how it functions, the more insight you'll have into your orgasms. With more insight, you will have more control; and with more control, you will invariably have more freedom and pleasure—and, ladies, isn't that what we're after?

But how do you move from that place of wanting an orgasmic experience but not being able to—for whatever reason—to the place of knowing your body well enough that, with the proper stimulation and a loving partner who wants to take you to another level, you can have an orgasm when you want one, how you want one, and where you want one? It's not surprising that a lot of women feel disappointed because they can't orgasm on a regular basis. Some women I've spoken to say they don't even know if they've ever had an orgasm. Other women are more certain and know they've never had an orgasm. Then there are men in the seminars who tell me that their wives or partners swear they've had orgasms but the men are certain they haven't. And I'm not talking about faking here; these women genuinely believe they have climaxed.

This book is intended to change all that. Many women (almost 70 percent) can't reach an orgasm through penetrative intercourse alone. This figure is based on the work of researchers from the University of Chicago who found that 22–28 percent of women in different age categories said they were unable to achieve orgasm during sex. May I say that if you are in this category you are not alone—*there is nothing wrong with you.* Most women can only climax on a consistent basis by clitoral stimulation (either manually or orally). And when you factor in how hectic our daily lives are, wedging in time for sex between appointments and alarm clocks, it's no wonder so many women and men feel dissatisfied with their sex lives and their ability to have good orgasms. As one woman said, "It used to be so good, even after the second baby was born. But now we are so tired and drained by the end of the day, we never even have sex anymore."

There may be some logic to why Wednesday night and Sunday morning are favorite times for sex for many couples. On Sundays, people often have more uninterrupted time together, and on Wednesdays, the midpoint of the week, people often need a distraction from work and everything else. Whatever the reason, the urge for pleasure is a positive one.

SECRET FROM LOU'S ARCHIVES

If, like most of us, what first got you interested in your partner was something emotional, then let your mind (remember, it's your largest sexual organ) do it again. A relationship is equal part intention and attention.

For most women, the reason for no or few orgasms with a partner boils down to two issues: (1) she isn't being stimulated in a way that works for her; (2) she is mentally not present. This is why it is often easier for a woman to be more easily orgasmic on her own, rather than with a partner: She knows exactly how to touch herself and is less distracted when she does so. And the same holds true for men.

HISTORICAL AND HYSTERICAL FACTS | The act of double penetration on a woman, one man penetrating vaginally and another anally, is known in France as "a sandwich à la Colette," thanks to the French novelist who supplied a detailed description of it in her novel.

Other women may be having difficulty because they haven't yet discovered the different types of stimulation that work for them, or they aren't comfortable touching their bodies. As I've said earlier, if a woman is not comfortable with self-pleasuring, then that's okay. She should just be honest with herself about how and why she might be having trouble orgasming.

Part of the problem or pressure surrounding orgasms is based on our so-called template of information that we've been taught (not that this is a classic subject learned in school) purporting that orgasms happen all the time, as if by magic. We've been led to believe this is true through movies, books, and magazines, which make having an orgasm seem effortless. Take for example, a recent book that promises every woman she can have a one-hour orgasm! Without reading the fine print, a woman might feel frustration and a sense of inadequacy when she discovers that her orgasms only last a few seconds or minutes. The more complete explanation uncovers that the orgasm that can last an hour requires all-over body stimulation that may keep a woman aroused, but certainly not at peak climax.

There are ways to improve the odds of having an orgasm, but most important is open, honest communication with your lover. You must explain to him what your preferences are. Believe me, he *wants* you to have an orgasm. No doubt, this will be more important to a man who is in love with you, but the truth is, even the most selfish man wants to know that he is capable of making it happen. If there's one thing I've learned in my years working with men in the sexuality seminars, it's that those men who feel they are skilled lovers connect their confidence to being able to please their women. I won't belabor this point, but the worst thing you can do for *either* of you is to fake it. That is the *ultimate* form of miscommunication. Why? Because men are "do machines," and if you give a man a signal that what he did worked well for you, he will immediately download that information onto his hard drive, and he will repeat the same series of actions at his next opportunity. So if you "fake it," he has unwittingly downloaded information that doesn't work. Now, where does that get either of you? As one man told me, "I don't care who a man is—if he gets his biggest turn-on from getting her on and off, he's the man! Any guy who puts himself first is giving her the bum's rush."

SECRET FROM LOU'S ARCHIVES

According to Joel Black and Susan Crain Bakos' book Sex Over 50, *the types of multiple orgasms are:*

➤ Compound singles—*where each orgasm is distinct and separated by a partial return to the resolution phase.*

➤ Sequential multiples—*orgasms occur two to ten minutes apart with minimal reduction in arousal between them.*

➤ Serial Multiples—*numerous orgasms are separated by mere seconds or minutes at most with no diminishment of arousal. Some women have this as one long orgasm with spasms of varying intensity.*

Variety Is the Spice of Life

Do you know that women can orgasm in at least ten different ways? As I say in *How to Give Her Absolute Pleasure*, I always like to encourage variety in all forms of sexual intimacy. My purpose in sharing this information with you is to let you know what is possible and, if you are interested, encourage you and others to push back the boundaries of self-imposed limitations to pleasure. I am *not* suggesting you have to do anything you do not want to. Like anything intimate, I want you to do only what you are comfortable doing. As with any buffet of ideas, sometimes we want merely hors d'oeuvres or dessert. Sometimes we long for the comfort-food entrée and sometimes we want the whole-meal deal. The following outlines what other women have experienced and shared, and I share it here with you.

There are ten ways or places in which women have experienced orgasm:

SECRET FROM LOU'S ARCHIVES

One of the more seductive things you can do for a man is let him know how much you are into what you are doing. Consider bringing your entire body into the experience as you move into position. Specifically, if you want to be in the female-superior position, rather than just sitting on his penis, start at the top of his head and move your whole body down him very slowly. Let him see, feel, and taste all of you as you make your way to his feet and then back up to his penis. The ladies in one seminar dubbed this the "Head-to-Toe F—" and attest to how sensual it is for both the man and the woman. As one man said, "There is no bigger turn-on for me. She gets me so hot when she does this, she drives me wild and makes me weak at the same time."

1. Clitoral
2. Vaginal and cervical
3. G-spot and AFE (anterior fornix erotic) zone
4. Urethral (U-spot)
5. Breast/nipple
6. Mouth
7. Anal
8. Blended/Fusion
9. Zone
10. Fantasy

Clitoral Orgasm

The clitoral orgasm is the most common and, for some women, the strongest orgasm; most women need some form of clitoral stimulation to orgasm. A clitoral orgasm occurs when the clitoris is stimulated to peak excitation. The sensation starts within the clitoral area and may radiate out from there. The nerve system involved is the pudendal nerve system, which is comprised of highly sensitive nerve fibers. Many women can attest to the highly sensitive nature of these nerves. The clitoris glans (the bud, so to speak) is the only visible part of a woman's clitoris. Until Dr. Helen O'Connell's paper was published in the *Journal of Urology* in 1998 ("Anatomical Relationship between the Urethra and Clitoris"), there was very little—if not zero—information about the actual, accurate size of a woman's clitoris in the mainstream press. Dr. O'Connell, a urological surgeon, discovered that the clitoris is actually ten times larger than had been previously reported. Most of the manufacturers of adult novelties (i.e., toys) are equally ignorant of the actual physiognomy of a woman's clitoris. Hence the majority of the products developed are not ergonomically functional.

| HISTORICAL AND HYSTERICAL FACTS | In 1930 there was a nude indoor bicycle race in Paris in which each woman's goal was to be the first to orgasm from rubbing on the seat. |

This has changed in recent years (see the illustration on p. 48), and thank heavens, for without understanding the size and dimension of this very important part of a woman's anatomy, how would we know how to activate all its pleasure signals?!

However, in terms of female orgasms, there has been a kind of clitocentrism for decades that has negatively impacted women's experience of their own orgasms. In other words, the sexologists of the day (Masters and Johnson in particular) promoted the idea that the clitoris and only the clitoris was the center of a woman's sexual universe. This idea made it seem that the only way a woman can orgasm is through clitoral stimulation. Thankfully psychologists Bernie Zilbergeld and Michael Evans offered an excellent critique of Masters and Johnson's work and pointed out the flawed manner in which Masters and Johnson's did their research and compiled their evidence and ideas. Now we know that though clitoral orgasms remain the most common, there are a wide variety of types to choose from and explore. Below I've outlined the main ways a woman can achieve a clitoral orgasm.

Manual Techniques for Clitoral Orgasm

Often manual stimulation of a woman is done while both of you are horizontal, but this position need not be your only option. Like dance steps, however, until you actually see how it can be done, it's hard to know how to move. In any position, the man should try to maintain good body contact, which is key to her pleasure. And his hands must be well maintained, no rough patches, with clean non-nibbled nails. If necessary, use water-based lubrication to ensure she doesn't dry out.

It's best, men, to rest the heel of your hand (and the wrist) to gently put pressure on her pubis mons, the area where the pubic hair starts. Be gentle and don't use too much pressure. You should feel the pubic bone underneath the base of your wrist—this will also help stabilize your arm. In other words, keeping it in the air will tire it out and affect overall mobility of your fingers. With your wrist anchored, you can deliver more of the gentle circles and back and forth motions that women prefer.

Circular and rocking palm hand motions also work well. If the man's penis is inside of her while he is touching her, he can try pulsing his PC muscle to make his penis jump. He can also use the index and middle fingers together in a straight up-and-down motion with the clitoral ridge and tip between the two of them. Often a woman uses this technique to stimulate herself.

VENUS BUTTERFLY

Illustrated is the two-hand position of the Venus Butterfly, and it is best done when a man is sitting up beside his partner. The term has an urban myth thing, which, to the best of my knowledge, is thanks to the creative minds of the writers of the '80s primetime soap *LA Law*. Although it was never disclosed on the show what the "VB" was, there have been many who have used the term, and here is a so-named manual "option" from the Schwartzs. The lower hand's thumb and fingers are cradling under her hips, resting on the surface of her body, neither are inserted, vaginally or anally. The upper active hand's middle finger will be doing as they describe the "bread-and-butter" stroke up and down over the clitoral area. The Schwartzs suggest imagining the middle finger to be a delicate butterfly wing. Be sure to use enough lubricant so she doesn't dry out and that the man's hands are smooth and his nails are trimmed.

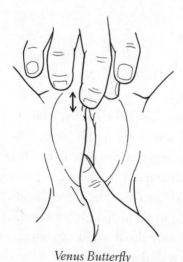

Venus Butterfly

IT TAKES THREE

Use three fingers held together curving over the labia; use the middle finger to stroke the clitoris and occasionally to slip inside the vagina. He can also use his index and ring fingers to squeeze the outer lips together from the outermost sides. Then he can do a short-range-of-motion with a front-to-back stroke and/or a squeeze, with a pulse up and down.

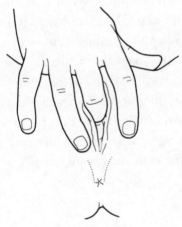

It Takes Three

Y-KNOT

For the Y-Knot move, the man spreads the labia with two fingers on one hand and, with the second hand on top, positions the middle finger, or two together, to massage the clitoris in a sideways, up and down, or circular motion. This move is great in that it doesn't tire the man's hands. She also has a nice "big" feeling when his hands are covering her, instead of just a finger. He may also want to try coming down on top: insert one finger inside and curve in and out of the vagina.

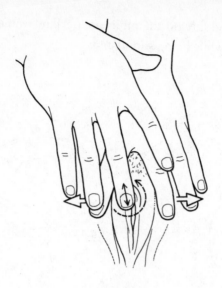

Y-Knot

THE SCULPTOR

The Sculptor move has two different styles—static and dynamic. The women in my seminars refer to both as the "take-me-home" moves. The man's hand is in the shape of a big "C." To orient his hand, imagine a clock over the woman's vulva and position his thumb to enter at six o'clock. There are a few critical things to remember with this: (1) the web of his hand should be between the thumb and forefinger, and the palm side knuckle area will be creating the sensation on the clitoris; (2) the inside edge of his inserted thumb can be putting pressure on the G-spot, and that sensation can be further heightened by using the other hand to press down on her abdomen in the pubic hair. The man should be able to feel the slight pressure on his thumb through the abdominal wall. Use a circular rocking motion with the "C" hand to spread the "C" fingers and put pressure on the pubis area. Many women enjoy pressure there while being stimulated.

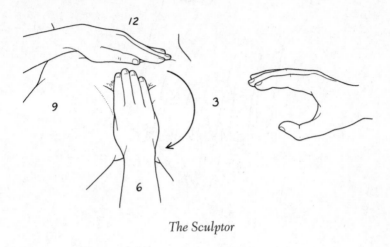

The Sculptor

Oral Techniques for Clitoral Orgasm

The power of a man's tongue on his lover cannot be underestimated—this warm, wet sensation can levitate most women. As one woman said, "There is nothing that compares to his mouth. It is softer, warmer, and he does so much more with it." Most women love cunnilingus because of the intensity of the physical sensation coupled with being able to relax into the sensation and do nothing—simply receive pleasure. For a number of women, this is a much more intimate form of sex than intercourse. "For me," one woman points out, "to let a man go down on me requires more trust."

Tongue motions include circular with the tastebud surface, up and down or back and forth with a broad tongue surface. Use either tongue surface, the top with tastebuds or the smooth undersurface. The combination of moves can create an endless variety of pleasure, but it's always best to start soft and build sensation gradually. If you need moves to make, trace the letters of the alphabet with your tongue. Also, be aware that the straight flicking with the tip of the tongue seen in adult films is not the move that really works. To start with, perhaps, but not for the entire run. So why the flicking-tongue scenes? If the films showed what really works they wouldn't have a shot.

If a man assumes a straight-on position between her legs and they are lying on the bed, he can get himself more comfortable by putting a pillow under her hips and one under his chest. That way, he's in a more comfortable position, his chin isn't squished against the mattress and his neck isn't scrunched. The best position is the classic. In this position, with the woman on her back, she can adjust the openness of her thighs and the intensity by adjusting her legs and holding herself open. If

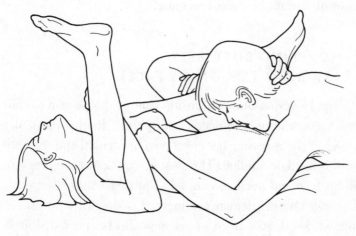

The Classic

she's in a chair the man simply needs to make sure he's comfortable too.

Some women are too sensitive to receive direct up-and-down clitoral strokes. If so, consider having her legs together or use only a downward stroke with your tongue. This way, the clitoral hood remains covering the highly sensitive glans. For women who prefer direct stimulation of the clitoris, the man needs to remember to lift the prepuce (or clitoral hood). Using the index and middle fingers of both hands, put upward pressure on the inside of the outer labia and lift the entire mons area or get her to hold herself open for you. You can also use pressure with a flat hand on her pubic mound and use a firm, upward (toward her head) pressure.

HOVERING BUTTERFLY
AKA SOMF (SIT ON MY FACE)

The Hovering Butterfly position allows the woman to control the sensation she needs and prefers. In this particular drawing, she is resting her chest on a headboard and the man has his head on a pillow. This way, he can adjust the pressure on his face and neck and not feel squished. After seeing this drawing, one gentleman commented, "My girlfriend arrives this weekend, so I need to get new sheets and I definitely need to buy a headboard."

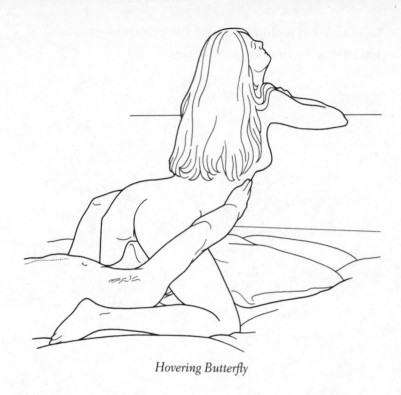

Hovering Butterfly

KIVIN METHOD

In the Kivin technique, the man is lying perpendicular to the woman. Her only responsibility is to receive sensation as she lies back. The man uses his tongue to stimulate his partner in a back-and-forth motion across the "K" points located on either side of the top and back of the clitoral hood. At the same time, he is maintaining contact on her "C" point (the perineum) with his fingertip so he can feel her preorgasmic contractions. (Those contractions are his guidepost that he is in the right place and making the right moves.) In the real-time video, where the demonstrations of this technique have not been edited, it is quite clear that the women experience rapid and intense orgasms in a short period of time.

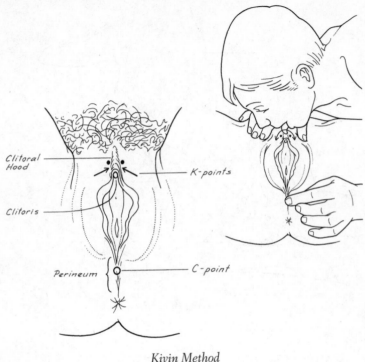

Kivin Method

Intercourse Techniques for Clitoral Orgasm

FEMALE SUPERIOR

A woman can experience an orgasm in the female-superior position, if she's already stimulated before getting on top of the man. This works for two reasons: (1) the woman has already been highly stimulated; and (2) she knows the clitoral sensations she needs to take her to orgasm and can create this

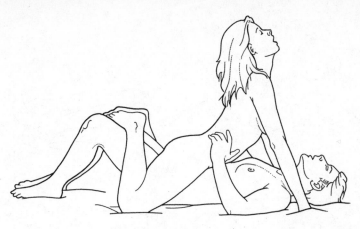

Female Superior

by a slow rocking or rubbing of her clitoral area on his shaft or pubis area. As soon as she's been clitorally stimulated to the point where her orgasm feels imminent, getting into the woman-superior position and starting to thrust will usually finish the job. It is a matter of precise timing. If she waits too long, she'll either reach orgasm before intercourse begins or lose the sensation altogether. As one woman put it, "We have to have the timing down or I come before when he is down on me, or I lose the edge when we change positions. But then sometimes it just works!"

MALE SUPERIOR

Women like the male-superior position because there is more body contact than in the other positions. While some of the others are perhaps considered more erotic, this one is the most romantic and connecting. Kissing and hugging are easily done in this position, and many women say it makes them feel

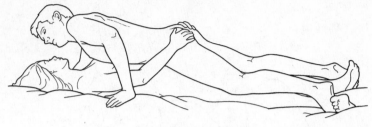

Male Superior

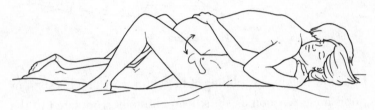

Male Superior, Coital Alignment Technique

safe and protected. "I am fairly tall," one woman explained, "and I love this position because my husband, who's even taller, makes me feel like a petite little flower. He covers all of me and that's the best."

In this position, the woman lies on her back with the man lying over her or slightly to the side of her. Men like this position because they can control the depth of penetration as well as the speed of the thrust. For some men, this is their tried-and-true way to have sex. As one man said, "I feel like I am the man. I know it isn't very PC of me, but it's just true."

A clitoral orgasm can also be achieved in this position using the CAT (coital alignment technique), which requires the man to penetrate deeply and to maintain constant motion and contact with her clitoris while he is deep inside of her.

This is a shallow stroke, unlike the typical large thrusting in-and-out motion of male-superior sex. In this position the clitoris is in direct contact with the base of his penis and it is the constant contact during up-and-down thrusting that does it. (See illustration on p. 227.) He can best achieve this position by having his shoulder up and over hers, while bracing his feet against a footboard, wall, or her feet. (See the illustration on p. 86.) This way he can rock against her clitoral area as he thrusts up and down. By maintaining constant contact with her clitoris, with the added stimulation of penetration, a woman can experience a deep, welling orgasm. As you can see, it's important that the man knows what he's doing here.

SIDE BY SIDE

Side by Side is a gentle, easygoing position that is conducive to orgasm. It is a position for partners who want the connection of insertion with little motion. It also good for those with hip or knee problems and when partners want to prolong their lovemaking. This is best for clitoral stimulation when the partners are facing each other. The woman can adjust the tightness at entry with her thighs, and then there is the ever so popular side-by-side spooning position.

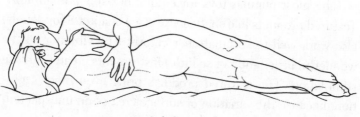

Side by Side

STANDING, SITTING, KNEELING

The standing, sitting, and kneeling group of positions work best if she is facing the man, especially if a chair is used. With

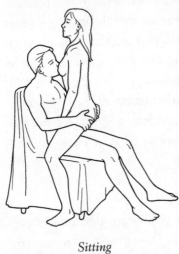

Sitting

her legs on either side, she can control the clitoral contact and motion she prefers. Standing is difficult to maintain if partners are differing heights. However, take a tip from young Russian lovers of the 1950s and '60s who, due to lack of privacy, often resorted to stairwells, and therefore used their differing heights to advantage. The woman stood on the stair above with her leg draped over the railing, while the man on the stair below enters her. (For this move, the woman would have to be wearing a skirt.) That way, they could hold on to each other and the railing for balance and leverage.

Toy Techniques for Clitoral Orgasm

The most popular toys for clitoral orgasms are vibrators. Textured products like shaft sleeves (see chapter 8 for details) also work well to stimulate her clitoris. The vibration of the wonderful little (and not so little) instruments creates intense stimulation. The textured products bring even more sensation, because the variation of surface creates an unexpectedness of feeling in the area.

Vaginal/Cervical Orgasm

The essential truth about vaginal/cervical orgasms is that they are not as precise as the other locations. The vaginal orgasm involves the barrel of the vagina as well as the cervix (the mouth of the uterus) and may involve even the uterus itself. There is a major physiological difference between clitoral stimulation and vaginal/cervical stimulation. With clitoral stimulation, there is an expanding and ballooning of the vaginal barrel and a lifting of the uterus back into the body, which prepares the vagina for the penis's entry. With vaginal stimulation, the uterus does not elevate. It pushes down into the vagina. As Dr. Herbert Otto says, "This orgasm takes place at the peak of stimulation of the vagina and cervix and expands from there. Sexologists Whipple and Perry call this process the A-frame effect."

With the approach of this orgasm there is a bearing-down effect and the vaginal opening becomes more relaxed. At the point of orgasm, it sometimes happens that the penis (or any object used for stimulation) is pushed out by the strength of these contractions. Also, the nerve systems that power the vaginal orgasm are the pelvic and hypogastic. This differs from the pudendal nerve system stimulated during clitoral orgasms. Hence it makes sense they would feel differently, because there are two different nerve systems being stimulated.

One woman described the vaginal orgasm in this way: "When my boyfriend gives me head, the orgasm has the sensation of pulling up and into myself. But when we do it doggy style, the orgasm has a much broader feeling. It seems to flow outside my body. It makes me want to arch and bear down."

Intercourse Techniques for
Vaginal / Cervical Orgasm

FEMALE SUPERIOR

Men tend to enjoy the female-superior position a lot. Not so much because the woman is doing most of the work, but because men, being visual creatures, love a good look at the front of her body. Not surprisingly, breast men like this position enormously; they love to see a woman's breasts move up and down with each motion she makes. As one man said, "I have to say this is my favorite position—even more because I love my wife's breasts."

SECRET FROM LOU'S ARCHIVES

The women who don't enjoy the female-superior position often say that its because they feel self-conscious about having their bodies exposed and in full view. If you don't feel particularly confident in the shape or tone of your body, it is understandable that you would feel funny about having it on display in this manner. But again, according to what men tell me, they are not looking at you with a critical eye at this time. Quite the contrary. Some men may be critical of women's bodies outside the bedroom, but during sex all women's bodies are beautiful to them. One man said this: "I am not having sex with her thighs. I am making love to all of her."

In the woman-superior position, the woman is usually straddling him with the bulk of her weight distributed evenly between both knees. The main motion that works is a back-

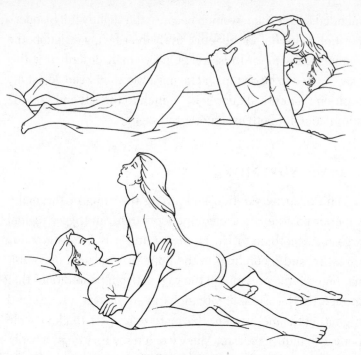

Female Superior

and-forth hip motion or circular screwing motion that allows the woman to stimulate her clitoris. A variation on this position, though somewhat difficult on the thighs, would be for the woman to squat over him with her feet flat on either side. Many women prefer the woman-superior position because it allows for deeper penetration. It also allows the woman to control the speed of the thrust since she is the person doing the thrusting. Having an orgasm may feel like more work on the woman's part than in the male-superior position, but many women find it to be well worth the effort. It is also a great position for having sex when the woman is significantly taller than the man.

According to Dr. Lasse Hessel, this position is recommended for pregnant women because the slightly full bladder's position helps buffer the fetus. In the rear-facing variation, the woman leans toward his feet. One woman described it this way: "I need to be on top and facing away, then I can adjust my position that critical quarter of an inch to the left and vary the stimulation for both my clitoris and vagina."

MALE SUPERIOR

The deep penetration and strong thrusting of the male-superior position are the components that can trigger vaginal orgasm. According to Dr. Herbert Otto, it is the continuous thrusting and "pounding" in the upper vaginal area in combination with the pressure in the vagina (from penetration) that induce the pleasurable vibrations in the cervix, uterus, and vagina. For some women, the mere entry of a thick or wide penis can induce orgasm. Many women say they enjoy a wider shaft because it "fills me up more." For other women, longer is better. These women have a highly sensitive area, "a rich plexus of sensory nerve endings" as noted by French physician

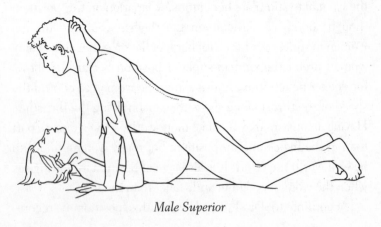

Male Superior

Gilbert Tordman in 1980, that is "next to the uterine cervix and vaginal cul-de-sac."

The same sensitive deep inner vaginal nerve plexus is noted by Dr. Barbara Keesling in her 1997 book, *Super Sexual Orgasm*. She says that "the key to the super sexual orgasm lies within a small passage of the vaginal canal, just beyond the cervix, known as the cul-de-sac. This small section of the vaginal canal is so extraordinarily enriched in sensitive nerve endings that in some women the slightest contact with a man's penis or sex toy can trigger instantaneous orgasm."

The position the woman holds her legs in will also vary the intensity of the angle and depth of penetration. The man can lift the lady to change the angle's intensity as well.

SIDE BY SIDE

A woman's orgasmic potential in the side-by-side position can vary greatly depending on her hormonal cycle. Often women are aware of differing points and areas of sensitivity in the vaginal wall, depending on where they are in their hormonal cycle, regardless of their age. Hence the position here

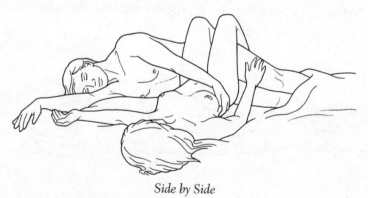

Side by Side

The Female Orgasm **95**

can be both restful and connecting but also effective in getting the man's penis to press against "just the right spot." (See "G-Spot" below for other side-by-side options.)

REAR ENTRY

According to Dr. Lasse Hessel, the rear-entry position gives women who have delivered vaginally an unexpected benefit. Since they have a more elastic vagina, the penis is able to stimulate more of the front wall. This is also very stimulating for the man, as the front of his glans is strongly stimulated by the angle with which he is entering her. It's as if he is almost thrusting between her cheeks. "There is something about rear entry that does it for me," one man from my seminars explained. "I think it is the feeling of so much of me up against her, and this includes my thighs against the back of hers."

STANDING, SITTING, KNEELING

In these more upright positions the woman is more able to adjust herself to stimulate the vaginal-wall area she prefers. Although it's possible to have a vaginal orgasm in this position,

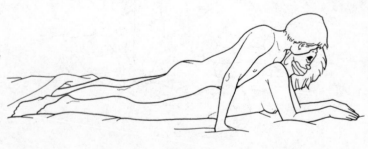

Rear Entry

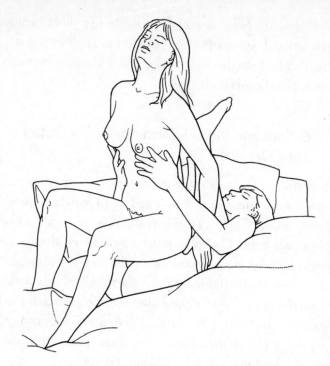

Sitting

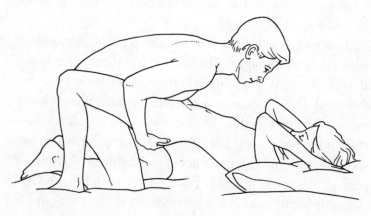

Kneeling

it is difficult because couples tend to use these positions as transitional, going from one position to another and not staying very long. In these particular styles, the man needs to have strong hip flexors and quads.

G-Spot and the AFE (Anterior Fornix Erotic) Zone Orgasm

Female orgasms during intercourse without direct clitoral stimulation are often associated with what is commonly known as the G-spot. The G-spot (named in honor of German physician Ernst Grafenberg, who first noted the tissue distinction) is an area approximately the size of a dime, located about two-thirds the length of your middle finger inside the vaginal entrance, above the pubic bone felt through the front wall (tummy side). When stimulated, the G-spot can enlarge to the size of a quarter. For some women, continuous stimulation can lead to a powerful orgasm. For others, G-spot stimulation is unpleasant. And just so you know, there are still other women for whom the much sought-after G-spot simply doesn't exist at all.

Ever since the G-spot was brought to public light in 1982 with the publishing of *The G-Spot* by Alice Kahn Ladas, Beverly Whipple, and John D. Perry, the G-spot has been controversial. Does it exist or not? Well, for some it does and is exceedingly pleasurable when stimulated, and for others, there is little or no sensation. This makes sense since this area above the anterior (tummy side) of the vaginal wall is considered to be vestigial tissue from genital evolution. Yet the G-spot is hardly new. It has been known to other cultures in the past since the first century A.D. The Chinese called this erotically sensitive area "the black pearl" and the Japanese referred to it as "the skin of the earthworm," and other people refer to it as the female prostate.

Not surprisingly, there are a number of misconceptions surrounding the G-spot. Dr. Beverly Whipple points out that the G-spot is not in the vaginal wall, but felt through it, and therefore requires more direct and firm pressure to stimulate it. Because of its position, many women have trouble finding their G-spot. The easiest way to locate it is when the woman is aroused enough so that the area is engorged with blood and can be felt more easily. Then, as Whipple suggests, the woman squats and reaches up inside of herself, as lying down isn't the easiest way to find it and often women's fingers are not long enough to reach the area. Another misconception involves female ejaculation. G-spot stimulation does not necessarily lead to ejaculation, though it can and has. But it's not required.

The AFE (anterior fornix erotic) zone is an area so named by Malaysian sexologist Dr. Chua Chee Ann. It is a spongy area of the vagina, and similar to the G-spot is located on the tummy side, but farther up the vaginal canal, closer to the cervix. Where as the G-spot is a defined area, the AFE is a longer, less defined area. However, the AFE responds to very gentle, light strokes, unlike the firm strokes used in G-spot stimulation. Citing his paper directly, Chua's study of 193 women in Malaysia stated that all but eleven "reported vaginal lubrication and increased erotic pleasure, and often orgasms, from stimulation of this zone." However, as Dr. Herbert Otto notes, this may be proportional to the number of women who can orgasm from G-spot stimulation, as Chua's population was very specific.

Manual Techniques for G-Spot and AFE Orgasm

Orgasm using manual techniques requires firm strokes in a come-here motion. This works best for the G-spot; AFE stimulation responds best to light, soft strokes.

Intercourse Techniques for G-Spot and AFE Orgasm

FEMALE SUPERIOR

In the female-superior position, a man can stimulate a woman if she is leaning back facing him or, as shown, facing

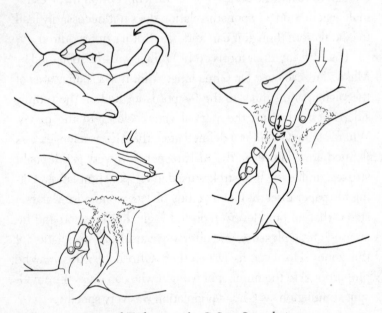

Manual Techniques for G-Spot Stimulation

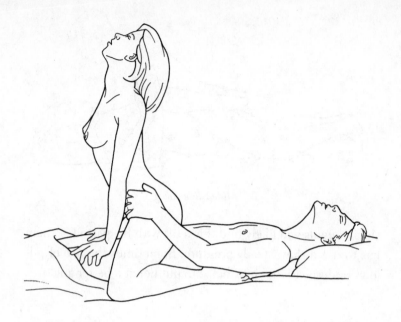

Female Superior

away; each of these alternatives helps to create an angle for his penis to move against the G-spot. The advantage of facing away from him is that the front of wall of the vagina (which would be the G-spot area) is stroked more firmly in this position, providing more direct stimulation to the G-spot area. Whether or not a woman can actually orgasm from G-spot stimulation, it is likely that you will find more pleasure with direct contact.

MALE SUPERIOR

Depending on the angle of his erection, the male-superior position can work. A gentleman lucky enough to have a prow-

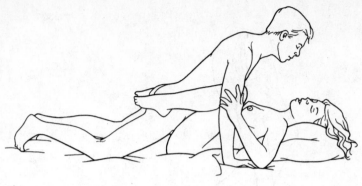

Male Superior

shaped penis will likely find this a hit with his partner. A man has to use a slow, steady pressure. Sometimes the use of pillows underneath her hips helps to put her at a better angle.

SIDE BY SIDE

In the side-by-side position, the woman usually has to be entered from behind and have her upper leg draped over her partner's. This enables him to have enough penetration range to reach the front vaginal wall firmly and consistently. Because

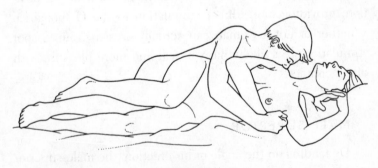

Side by Side

this position has a limited range of motion, the man is able to maintain better contact and the woman can adjust the pressure on the front wall by flexing her hips back or raising her leg.

REAR ENTRY

Rear entry is especially good for women who have delivered vaginally since their nerve pathways are more "alert" and sensitive to receiving stimulation because the vaginal barrel is more flexible and the penis can hit the right spot more easily. Keep in mind that a woman kneeling on all fours can lower her shoulders to heighten the pressure angle.

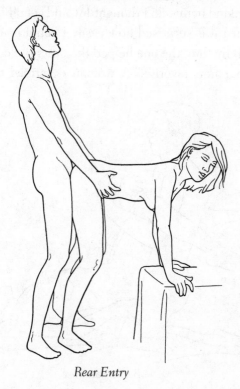

Rear Entry

STANDING, SITTING, KNEELING
AKA THE BTS POSITION (BETTER THAN SEX)

The "BTS" position allows a man to remain kneeling or standing while he enters his partner at a 90-angle. She is lying faceup on the bed and then places her heels on his shoulders or her knees into the crook of his elbows. In either position she can easily adjust to her preferred angle. He now is able to show off his gym work by flexing his arms. By further pulling up the woman's hips, he greatly increases the pressure stroke along the G-spot area. "I could watch her all day when I do this. Her breasts jiggle, she arches her back and gets that flush around her neck. I thought I would get off balance doing this, but I was surprised how easily I could maintain my hip and arm rhythm, the one helped the other build . . . it has become our new favorite." A woman described the sensation

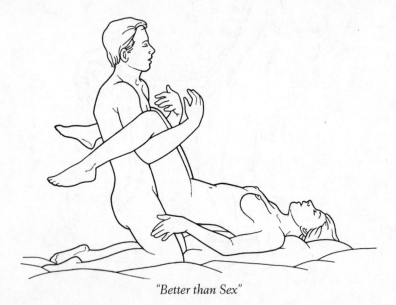

"Better than Sex"

this way: "The first time he did this I almost went out of my mind. There was a build-up of heat unlike I'd ever felt. But I need to be careful because depending on my cycle, sometimes I am too sensitive and it becomes sensory overload. But when it works, Girlllll!"

U-Spot/Urethral Orgasm

Like the clitoris, stimulating the urethra is also very pleasurable for some women, which makes sense since the urethra (and its paraurethral glands) is surrounded on three sides by the clitoris and is located between the clitoral glans and the vaginal opening (introitus). So the urethra, where urine exits a woman's body, is just below the clitoris and above the vaginal entry. You may recall from the Dr. Helen O'Connell diagram (page 48) that the clitoris is much larger than meets the naked eye, which is an indication of how stimulating it can also stimulate the urethra.

Manual Techniques for U-Spot Orgasm

Some women have said they enjoy firm manual pressure on their urethral area when masturbating. Due to the small area involved, in order to concentrate the sensation in the right place, it's necessary to use refined circular or up-and-down pressure strokes.

Oral Techniques for U-Spot Orgasm

One technique described to me was for him to apply strong and constant pressure on the urethral area using his lower lip wrapped over his teeth during oral sex. A woman's partner can also open her inner labia to expose the urethral area and use a soft gentle tongue stroke right on it. Her reaction will let you know right away whether she likes it.

Intercourse Techniques for U-Spot Orgasm

FEMALE SUPERIOR

Orgasm in the female-superior position is possible, especially if the woman is leaning strongly forward with her legs widely spread to get as much of the top vaginal entry area in contact with the base of the man's shaft.

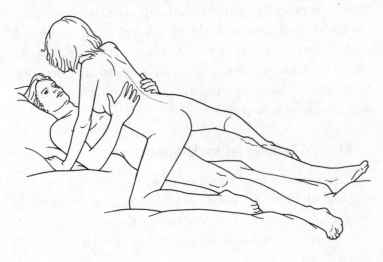

STANDING, SITTING, KNEELING

It is possible to orgasm in a standing, sitting, or kneeling position if the man uses short strokes and the woman has her legs wrapped around him, pulling herself in closely.

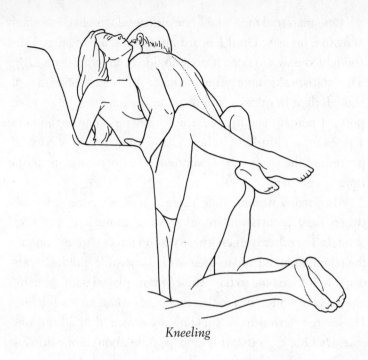

Kneeling

Breast/Nipple Orgasm

Breast and nipple orgasms are apparently much more common than you might think. Dr. Herbert Otto describes the breast orgasm as happening at the peak of stimulation when the sensation seems to radiate from the breasts. He claims (and supports) that it is the second most common form of orgasm among women, which seems especially true of women from our grandmothers' and mothers' generations. Women of an earlier time were much more likely to be afraid to "go all the way" because of the moral restrictions of their time or a fear of getting pregnant. Instead they enjoyed a lot of heavy "petting" and "necking" sessions in which they had breast or nipple orgasms.

One man told me, "I had one girlfriend who had extremely sensitive breasts. Until I heard about a breast orgasm, I just thought she was making it up. I couldn't touch them enough." The statistics support the evidence of breast orgasms, although their frequency is in dispute: Masters and Johnson report a 1 percent occurrence; the Kinsey report gives the same 1 percent, and in Dr. Herbert Otto's study group of 513, 29 percent of the women had experienced a breast orgasm at one time or another.

Also, many women state there is a direct connection between their breasts and nipples being stimulated and their genitals. For other women, there was no direct connection, but the stimulation did add to their overall orgasmic build. For others, it is bothersome to have their breasts played with. Nursing mothers have often experienced orgasms when breast-feeding. These are referred to as suckling orgasms and in all but one case, Dr. Otto cites that this kind of stimulation during nursing was accompanied by uterine, vaginal, or cervical contractions.

Manual Techniques for Breast/Nipple Orgasm

In the case of manual stimulation, use whatever works for the woman. Some women want soft, full circles, and some women want you to bite or pinch their nipples. The rule of thumb here is the more intense sensation is best done after lots of stimulation.

Oral Techniques for Breast/Nipple Orgasm

Whether it is a constant suction or a suction in combination with nibbles, or licks, or tongue strokes, the sky is the limit with how you can stimulate breasts orally. If you're not sure what she likes, ask her to suck on your tongue or lips to show how much suction she wants on her nipples.

Toy Techniques for Breast/Nipple Orgasm

There are products on the market now that can apply direct suction and vibration to the breasts and nipples. Nipple clips have been around for a long, long time and should be used judiciously. A basic rule of thumb should be to never leave anything on someone's body too long (numbness is the warning sign) or you risk causing permanent nerve damage, which is hardly the aim of sex toys.

Mouth Orgasm

If we understand that as babies we experience our entire universe through our mouths, then maybe it's not as hard for us to imagine actually experiencing an orgasm through our mouths. Women have reported experiencing these starting in the lips and spreading out, and they would often be triggered by stimulation of lips, tongue, roof of the mouth, and the throat—*without any genital stimulation*. Some women experience a mouth orgasm through kissing or while giving oral sex to a man. Other women describe the sensation as a whole body orgasm accompanied by uterine and vaginal contractions.

When I first asked a seminar group if they had ever been with someone who had had a mouth orgasm, one man looked at me like I had five eyes, and another man looked taken aback and said softly, "Yeah, yeah I did." According to Dr. Herbert Otto's research, of his 205-member research group, 20 percent had experienced a mouth orgasm. They do exist.

The best technique is great, long kissing. Use more lip play, sucking on the lips. Dr. Mantak Chia suggests taking your partner's upper lip into your mouth and running your tongue along the inside of the upper lip. One woman reported, "I don't know what he did, but he did this tongue thing and my knees buckled. I then asked him to do it again. Same result. I think it was all in the lip sucking."

Anal Orgasm

If we understand how sensitive our lips can be . . . it's not too hard to imagine how sensitive the other end of our gastrointestinal tract may be. I like to think of anal play as the new frontier—similar to how oral sex used to be treated before it too became "normal" instead of associated with things "dirty." One thing I've noticed in the past few years of giving seminars

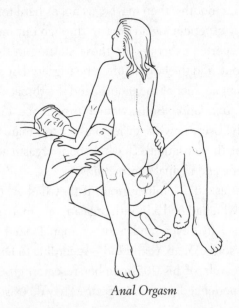

Anal Orgasm

is that more and more women and men are asking questions about anal sex. Now you can take this as a gentle suggestion to try or not—your body, your choice. However, the women and men who have added this option to their sexual repertoire say it can create more fun, spice, and often a lot of sexual pleasure.

Women have to be comfortable being penetrated, so I suggest first using a clean, well-lubricated finger to test the waters. Once she is more open and begins to respond to the stimulation, you can experiment with other playthings (see below).

There is a physiological reason anal penetration can be difficult: There are actually two anal sphincters—one under voluntary control, so you can consciously relax it, and another under involuntary control, which requires dilation with a finger or toy to be relaxed.

Manual Techniques for Anal Orgasm

Any manual sensation that you think your partner would like on his or her lips, they are likely to enjoy anally. Use gentle stroking, outlining the area, and soft entry.

Oral Techniques for Anal Orgasm

Be sure you know your partner's hepatitis status before having unprotected anal sex, aka anilingus. (You might want to keep this in mind for any place you kiss.) The best techniques are tongue flicking or sucking, or a combination of the hand and mouth.

Toy Techniques for Anal Orgasm

Be sure that the toy you use for anal sex has a flange (an enlarged base) so that it can't inadvertently slip inside the rectum by mistake. Because the PC muscles encircle the anus, when it contracts during an orgasm, you can also feel it through vaginal and urethral orgasmic contractions in women and urethral and anal in men. If you insert something anally it gives the PC muscle something to contract against, and with more resistance comes more sensation. Anal beads can also heighten the orgasmic response by being pulled out all at once or sequentially at the moment of orgasm. Those who enjoy them say they create an additional "orgasmic wave."

Be sure not to share these toys and don't use a toy both anally and vaginally—even if you've really cleaned it.

Blended, or Fusion, Orgasm

The blended orgasm, as named by Whipple and Perry in 1982, is when more than one area of the body is stimulated at the same time, increasing the overall intensity and expanding the orgasmic sensation. As an example, stimulation of the clitoris becomes greater when combined with breast or G-spot stimulation. This is understandable since we know from research that the two areas are enervated by the two separate nerve systems—the pudendal for the clitoris, and the pelvic for the G-spot. With more nerves involved, there is more (broader) sensation.

Zone Orgasm

A zone type of orgasm is much more individualistic because it occurs in various parts of people's bodies that are rarely associated with stimulation to orgasm. For example, people—both men and women—have experienced orgasms from having their necks licked or their fingers sucked, or their thigh/groin area stroked.

Fantasy Orgasm

A fantasy orgasm is described as the ability to orgasm by fantasy alone—with no genital stimulation. Suffice it to say that this is likely the one type of orgasm that most people would like to be able to create at will, and there are probably only a chosen few who can. It differs from fantasy aiding and abetting orgasms, which in general is a most common practice. Fantasy orgasm was documented in the lab in 1992 by Whipple, Ogden, and Komisaruk, and showed that the body's physiological response to an imagery-induced orgasm was no different from one induced by physical stimulation. The same increase in blood pressure, heart rate, pupil diameter, and pain threshold were reported.

Sex for One

Masturbation is referred to euphemistically in any number of ways: self-pleasuring, dating oneself, twiddling the twinkle, and frigging, to name just a few. For most women, similar to men, masturbation is the way they learn to orgasm first, and therefore most easily. Self-pleasuring is about discovering yourself in a private, safe environment. When you get to know your body, you enable yourself to feel more pleasure. You can show your partner how to touch and stimulate you, and you may even discover that your partner wants to share this experience with you.

We know that women can and will talk just about anything, but here is one area where detail is often omitted. We might share that we used an X, Y, or Z vibrator, or refer to the time in front of the Jacuzzi jet, but the details are never revealed. Yet 70 percent of women say they masturbate. Why the discomfort? The discrepancy? I presume women are still socially conditioned to refrain from experiencing sex as pleasure as a way to repress their power. This would also apply to self-pleasuring.

Of comfort to us all is that again our sexual individuality shows through in our masturbatory preferences. "No two women have been observed to masturbate in identical fashion," notes Masters and Johnson. This observation is repeated by Dr. Fithian's research that came up with the idea of "orgasmic fingerprinting" to underscore the unique nature of everyone's orgasmic response patterns.

Techniques

MANUAL

➤ Some women enjoy a soft circular motion, starting at the top of the mons and circling gently until they are inside the inner labia, and then back out again.

➤ Another technique is to use two or three stiff fingers either on top of the outer labia in a circular motion to stimulate the clitoral ridge underneath or, with lubricated fingers, stimulate the clitoral ridge itself.

When using a lubricant, make sure to use one that is water-based, as oil can cause a yeast or bladder infection.

➤ A single finger, usually the middle, on the clitoris in the up-and-down stroke while holding the outer labia open with the index and ring fingers.

➤ Combine an inserting stroke of two fingers with a circular, up-and-down, or a swift back-and-forth stroke over the top of clitoral glans area in varying pressure.

➤ Combine with nipple stimulation for more sensation.

➤ Some women will use the fingertips of their "free" hand to apply pressure on the line from their belly button down to the top of the pubic mons. This helps to build sensation in a broader area.

➤ Some women enjoy a light tapping on the head of the clitoris when they are already stimulated.

WATER

➤ Fill the tub with a few inches of your preference of hot or warm water and then place your genitals directly under the flow of water. A sticky bath mat on the bottom of the tub will anchor you so that you can use a small rocking motion to heighten the buildup.

➤ Use your hands to hold yourself open more, and expose more surface of the genital area to sensation. The more taut the skin is, the greater the sensation you can create.

➤ Bidets can also work their magic—especially the type that has a central fountain spurt.

➤ Handheld showerheads have become many women's best friend—try it in the morning!

> In the Jacuzzi, position yourself over the jet. Some women find it more intense when the jet is streaming from behind, which makes sense as the water is forcing the clitoral hood up and exposing more of the clitoral shaft, one of the most sensitive parts of you, to the water jet.

> Some women say they can fantasize more in water because they are better able to disconnect from the world.

USING SURFACES

> Some women enjoy riding a pillow or rubbing against a particular fabric, which they often learned to do as young girls, quite by accident.

> A porcelain sink: this idea came from a woman who told me, "I used to lean against those big old porcelain sinks at school. I was very tall so I'd position myself against the edge and rock until I came. I did it for years. Everyone just thought I liked to have clean hands."

> A man's leg: "I can come just rubbing against my husband's thigh."

VIBRATORS

Women tend to fall into two categories when it comes to vibrators: they either prefer the direct clitoral stimulation of a smaller vibrator or a broader, more general sensation of a larger vibrator such as the Hitachi Magic Wand.

> With the smaller vibrator, the action is often a cycle of touches until there is enough buildup and then

the clitoris can tolerate more direct stimulation. Often women will position the vibrator against the fleshy outer labia to cushion the intensity. And with this placement it is impacting more of the long clitoral leg. Some women find that direct clitoral contact with a vibrator is way too intense. One woman said, "I love a slow buildup and I felt like my orgasm got pulled out of me with a vibrator; it was too much."

➤ With a broader-head vibrator, such as the Hitachi, there is more displacement of vibration and sensation. To diffuse the sensation if it is too intense women can use a washcloth or a piece of clothing against the head of the wand to cushion or buffer the labia. Some women enjoy placing their wand on a pillow then lying on top of it and using a pelvic thrusting motion in combination with the vibration.

➤ For those who might want to get to another level entirely, women suggest trying a Sybian vibrator, which is ridable and can be used solo or with a partner. It is, however, very large and expensive.

While women can attest to experiencing orgasms in at least ten different ways, most of us tend to come in the most familiar (and the easiest) way possible. If you want to spice up your sex life, stretch your boundaries a bit, and you don't mind taking perhaps more time to play around with your honey, then I suggest you sample one of the types that appeals to you. By combining one, two, or three of these techniques, who knows what will happen. Mother Nature gave us bodies and imaginations: Be sure to use them both.

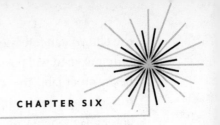

The Male Orgasm

*How to Get the Most
from the Tools You've Got*

The X-Y Difference

T he male orgasm differs from the female orgasm in numerous ways. First, whereas women can experience an orgasm in at least ten different ways, men generally experience
an orgasm in one of four main ways: (1) stimulation of their
penis (usually accompanied by ejaculation) either manually,
orally, or through intercourse; (2) via the prostate or the anus;
(3) through stimulation of the nipples; and (4) for a lucky few,
through fantasy, without any physical stimulation at all. This,
of course, makes sense since most men have experienced wet
dreams, which may very well be Mother Nature's way of getting rid of excess sperm production.

These four types indicate *where* orgasm is usually stimulated, but they don't give the whole sense of *how* men have orgasms. The key to understanding how you can have a better orgasm (i.e., experience more pleasure and control) is through awareness: awareness of your body, its muscles, and its nerve endings. Wherever or however an orgasm occurs, men tend to experience orgasms in terms of physical intensity and/or emotional connection. Sometimes you and your partner may "just want to have fun," in which case you're more focused on physical intensity. If you are in a more romantic mood, feeling very close to each other, you may be making love in order to increase the feeling of emotional closeness. In this way, you're using sex as a vehicle for emotional connection.

As we saw, the four stages of arousal are a helpful way of getting the "big picture" of what is happening during sex. But as noted, men and women are often on different schedules, with women taking longer to become aroused but staying aroused longer. On the other hand, men have a quicker response to stimulation, but generally a shorter arousal period.

SECRET FROM LOU'S ARCHIVES

More often than any other position, the partner on top is going to have better control of the orgasm due to them having better control of thrusting.

What I've gathered below are the seven different ways men can orgasm. Try these singly or in combination and you might just discover a new path to pleasure. I also recommend that both of you read this section together so you can share what interests and excites you.

The Types

There are essentially seven different ways that a man can experience an orgasm:

1. Intercourse
2. Manual
3. Oral
4. Prostate and anal
5. Fantasy
6. Nipple/breast
7. Toys

Intercourse Orgasm

Yes, most men (and women) think the penis is the lightning rod of male orgasm. Of course, for most men it is the part of the anatomy that first introduced them to the power of and the pleasure of their sexuality, through masturbation (albeit done quickly, so Mom wouldn't catch you). It's my hope that once you cover the material that follows, you will see there can indeed be expanded horizons of experience for you. For some it will be the discovery that the stimulation of another area enhances penis-located orgasms. You will learn how to take your pleasure to another level, so to speak. Others of you will find yourself crossing into new territory, experiencing orgasms from other places in your body—beyond the nipples, for instance. You may find that when your lover rubs your feet, you find yourself aroused . . . who knows?!

HISTORICAL AND HYSTERICAL FACTS	Here are a few orgasms I hadn't heard of before: eyegasm (maintain eye contact during sexual orgasm) and Jellogasm (if your normal physical response is all-over body tension, try letting your entire body be like Jell-O).

I have outlined below the main positions men use to have orgasms through intercourse. These positions are accompanied by information that will help give you a sense of how to access a certain feeling or increase intensity.

FEMALE SUPERIOR

Many men love when the woman is on top "riding high." Given that the majority of men are very visual, it makes sense that this would be a favored position, and especially for breast men, who can watch the motion of her breasts. After all, from a "work" standpoint, the man doesn't need to do much other than watch the show, because he knows that she is doing what works for her.

The position in the center illustration on page 122 is good when a man is much larger than the woman and they want to experience as much tactile closeness as possible. In this position, a man can even practice exercising those gym-developed abs by pressing up and lifting his partner at the same time. As

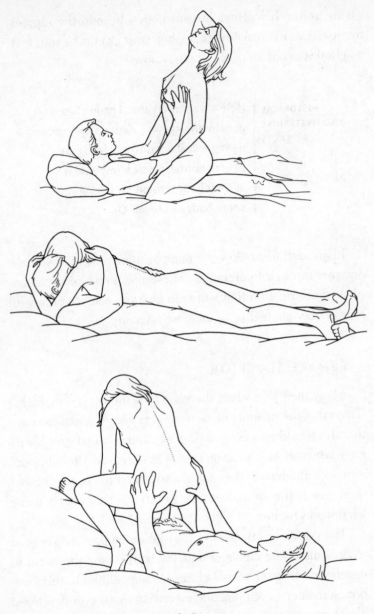

Female Superior

a result of these variations, some men say they are aroused more quickly in this position. Muscle tension has been known to assist orgasmic sensation. They can relax into receiving sensation and climax more easily. Note her feet on his for ease in thrusting.

An alternative to this position is "Chinese style," the illustration shown at the bottom of page 122, where a man who loves a rear view can watch not only the insertion of himself inside of her, but also his partner's buttocks.

MALE SUPERIOR

The male-superior position, of course, is referred to traditionally as "missionary style," apparently named thusly because so many South Sea natives witnessed this position by Christian missionaries sent over to convert them. Sometimes the predictability of this position (like a favorite comfort food) allows a man to relax into his orgasm in a natural, accustomed way. Whether this is "normal" or "regular" for you, this position invariably ends up being one of the more popular with women because they are enveloped by their man. As I often hear from women, it "gives me a feeling of safety." And "it feels so male."

In the top illustration on page 124 he is inserted most deeply, and in the center illustration there is deep penetration with close clitoral contact.

For added stimulation, a man's partner may want to try the Florentine method, as seen in the bottom illustration on page 124, of holding his penile skin gently but firmly at the base of the shaft with a ring of her forefinger and thumb to intensify the sensation for him. It's well worth the practice to get this down.

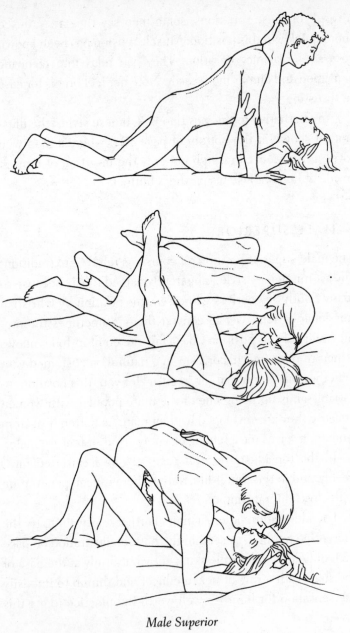

Male Superior

SIDE BY SIDE

There is a reason why spooning, as seen below, is a preferred position for many couples. This position not only provides a good, strong emotional connection, it also is restful.

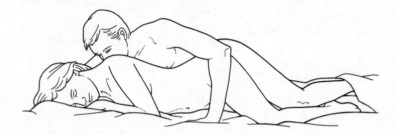

Now it can also be much more athletic, as shown in the illustration below and also on page 126, if you are motivated, and then after some time, become restful again. If you've tried other

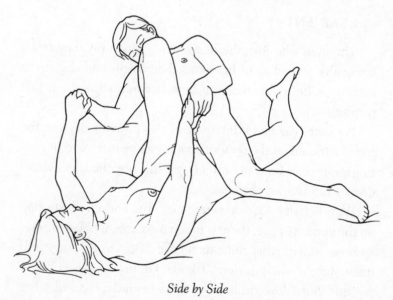

Side by Side

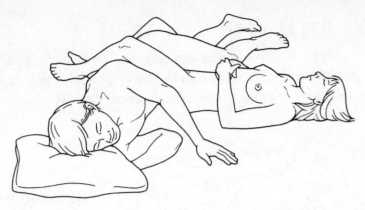

Side by Side

positions during one lovemaking session and you end up here, after coming, you both may fall into a tranquil, satisfied sleep, as in this classic position.

REAR ENTRY

The men who love the rear-entry position say they relish being able to feel all of her along their thighs and abdomens with their flesh "bouncing against her buttocks . . . it just turns me on."

For both, the erotic intensity of this position, seen in the top illustration on the opposite page, can be increased by putting a mirror in front of both of you; this way the sheer visual display can turn up the heat.

With her shoulders lowered, as in the bottom illustration on the opposite page, there is much more intense glans stimulation as well as what some men have shared as the more animal nature of the position: "I know I'm not supposed me to say this, but I love drilling her from behind." For still other

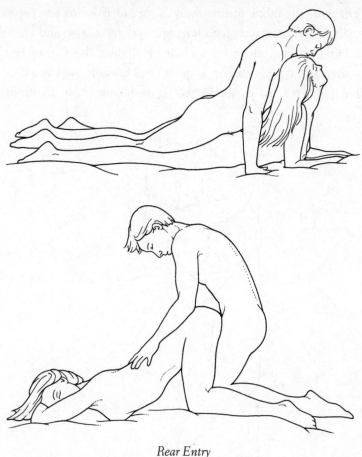

Rear Entry

men who love this position, they get into the scent of sex that comes from this proximity to her genitals.

STANDING, SITTING, KNEELING

Couples often use the standing, sitting, and kneeling variations as starting or transitional positions—they are good for changing the momentum (always a nice idea during sex, especially if you have time for a long lovemaking session and enjoy adding variety). Be it on a chair or pillows, the two of you seated as a couple can be as quiet or as boisterous as you prefer. However, as we see in the figure below, these positions

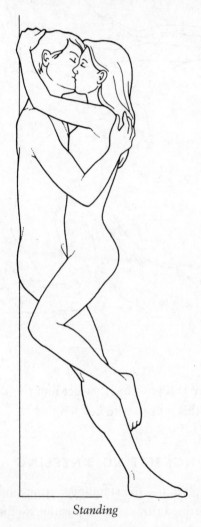

Standing

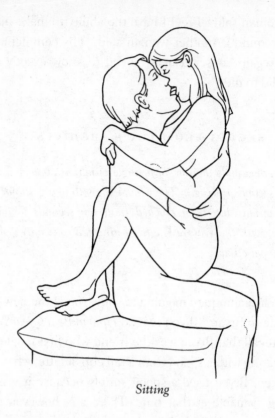

Sitting

tend to be difficult to maintain long enough for orgasm, for even the most athletic of us. Take a tip from men's magazines and do not overlook the benefit of possibly working out specific muscle groups while holding her and maintaining a standing or squatting position.

Manual Orgasm

Manual stimulation of the penis deserves its own category, because having your lover use her hands to arouse and bring you to orgasm gives both of you enjoyment—double your fun!

As one woman said, "I feel I have the ability to make him go out of his mind." Another woman said, "His comment was, 'When I regain consciousness I need to know exactly what you just did to me.'"

SECRET FROM LOU'S ARCHIVES

The average male orgasm for a single climax is about ten to fifteen seconds in length. The woman's length of orgasm for a single climax has been clocked from ten seconds to one minute, with the average length of nineteen to twenty-eight seconds per climax.

The first technique I'm going to show you is the now infamous "Ode to Bryan." If you've read *How to Be a Great Lover*, you may recall that Bryan was the friend who first taught me, demonstrating with a spoon from a tall cup of latte, what feels best to men. Bryan used a spoon simply because it was the only thing available at that time. There are, however, more suitable items on which to hone your skills. In the seminar we use an "instructional product," my professional term for a Doc Johnson Realistic dildo with a suction cup at the base.

These instructions are geared for women to do for their men. They are based on the demonstrations I give to women in the sexuality seminars. However, for your purposes, you and your partner can practice on the "real thing" (i.e., his penis) or use a dildo or a cucumber. Some women have tried using bananas, but the results were disappointing—bananas are not nearly firm enough.

ODE TO BRYAN
(AKA THE PENIS SAMBA)

Step 1. Apply a lubricant of your choice generously to both hands. It's a good idea to warm it slightly by rubbing your hands together.

Step 2. Start with your hands out in front of you, palms facing away and thumbs down. Your thumbs are held against your index finger, they are *not* pointing down like little spikes. With one hand (it doesn't matter which one you start with), gently but firmly hold the base of the penis. Your view should be of the back of your hand and four fingers. Your wrist should be cocked forward toward his body. His view will be of your thumb, nestled into his pubic hair. Position your other hand so that it will be ready to move into position (it can be resting on his thigh or testicles) once the first hand's stroke is complete. When you have completed one "cycle" both hands typically will be in constant motion, so you need not worry about where they will rest. They won't be.

Step 3. Maintain placement of your hand while stroking up the shaft in a single continuous motion.

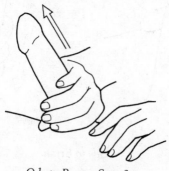

Ode to Bryan, Step 3

Step 4. When you get to the head, rotate your hand slightly as if you were carefully opening a jar. Do not rotate your hand *until* you reach the head. Bryan's comment was, "*The twist is the most critical part. Don't do it until you get to the top.*"

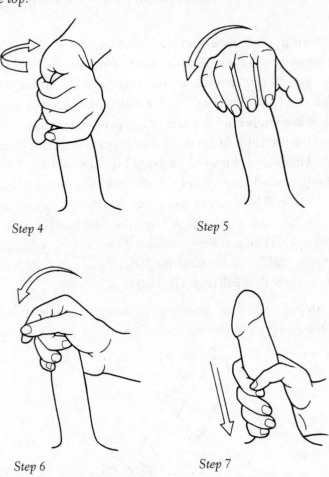

Step 4

Step 5

Step 6

Step 7

Ode to Bryan

Step 5. Maintaining as much contact as possible between the head of the penis and the palm of your hand, rotate your hand over the top of the penis, as if you were sculpting it's head with the entire palm of your hand.

Step 6. Because of the rotation (aka the twist), your thumb will now be facing you and the back of your hand will be facing him. Come down the shaft again firmly to the starting position and immediately move your second hand into starting position, on top of your finishing hand. The starting hand just slides into position over the top of the finishing hand to maintain motion. Note: This is important because you want to have a continuous flow of sensation. You'll get into a flow of motion very quickly.

Step 7. Follow steps 2–6 immediately with your other hand. Alternate hands repeatedly until . . .

Penis Samba is **Ode to Bryan** done very quickly and *only* at the top/head. And, as you will no doubt discover, this move takes on a rhythm all its own. You will create a ring with the index finger and thumb of one hand just below the head of his penis to create a mini lifesaver ring. This enables you to concentrate all the sensation in the first $1^{1}/_{2}$ inches of his penis—the most sensitive area for most men. With your other hand, move your hand on the head of his penis in a circular motion (imagine you have ink in your palm and you are trying to apply an even coat on the head of his penis). Once you finish the application, switch hands and repeat the motion with your other hand.

BASKET WEAVE

Basket Weave is another seminar favorite. Not only does it do wonders all on its own, it is the motion that makes giving him a Pearl Necklace (page 198) the "bomb."

Step 1. Apply your lubricant of choice generously to both hands.

Step 2. Clasp your hands together, interlacing fingers.

Step 3. Relax thumbs in order to make hole.

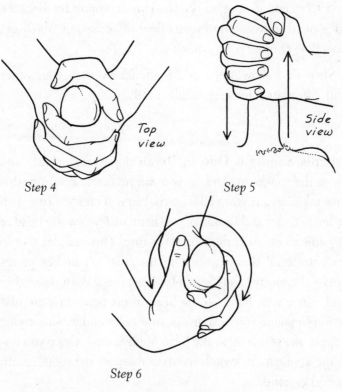

Basket Weave

Step 4. Lower your clasped hands onto his penis. The fit should be snug, much like a tight vagina. In essence you are creating an impostor vagina.

Step 5. Move your clasped hands up and down the shaft, continuing the firm and gentle hold.

Step 6. Twist your clasped hands slowly as they go up and down the shaft, much like the motion inside a washing machine. Gently, however, as this isn't a quick swishing back and forth. Coordinate an up-and-down move with a gentle twisting stroke.

Oral Orgasm

Men love, love, love to orgasm orally! So how do we bridge the gap with this very real men's pleasure and some women's hesitation or disinclination to do this for their man? In all the years I've been doing seminars and speaking to women about their sexual experiences, I've found that there is one obvious distinction between those women who *enjoy* performing oral sex on their lovers and those who don't. The difference is that the women who do enjoy giving oral sex know they are giving him something very special and it is a huge turn-on for them to know "I can make him feel that amazing." The women who don't like to give oral sex often feel they "have to" or are "supposed to do it" and therefore resent it and find the concept unpleasant.

As with any experience in life, if the first encounter a woman has with oral sex, or any sex for that matter, is positive she will likely maintain a positive attitude about it. However, as in life, there are many different ways of reacting to any event and sometimes we encounter partners who are less than deserving or gentle when we are learning or trying something new. Until we have the reaction of a supportive and sensitive partner, we don't know or have confidence of how we are as a lover, as our partners are our litmus test on whether we are good or bad. And often men, and women as well, do not know how to guide their partners even when they ask, and that makes sense too. How can one not know? Easy. The analogy I use to explain it is this: Remember when you are having a massage you are not concentrating on what is being done to your body; your job is to relax and feel. So when you are with a partner, your job is not to *analyze* what he or she is doing, your job is to feel.

Women are like horses: you can lead them to water but do not expect them to drink—they will do so in their own time, if they so choose. I just heard of a hilarious website selling CDs with subliminal messages supposed to make women perform oral sex. How do you spell scam on the Net? Rather than a CD to manipulate her mind, why not be straight up and deliver the kind of attention that turns her head—that will give a man more access than any CD.

HISTORICAL AND HYSTERICAL FACTS	A recent survey of prostitutes revealed that the most frequently requested sex is fellatio.

However, there is a way for a woman to begin to enjoy this most intimate of sexual pleasures with her man. The secret to a woman's success and enjoyment is in taking *control*. As one man told me, "When she takes me into the back of her throat, first it is so hot just watching her do it and then when she swallows on the head of my cock it is like there are a hundred little fingers running all over it—as if there were three women in bed with me."

Oral sex is not only more fun for the man when he doesn't have to work at it, it's also a lot more fun for the woman that way, too. Some of the reasons I hear over and over again as to why women don't like giving oral sex is that they gag when the penis gets to the back of their mouths, they are asked to deep-throat, or they don't want to start what they don't want to swallow. Make no mistake, giving a man oral sex is very much an acquired skill—even though it does exist in the animal kingdom. About gagging, Mother Nature gave us a gag reflex as a way of keeping our throats protected. The gag reflex was incorporated into human biology for safety purposes. So chances are you're going to gag when performing oral sex—most women do. So don't worry if it doesn't come naturally or immediately.

Also the Ring and Seal technique will take care of how to handle the gag reflex. Your index finger and thumb on whichever hand you use the most are attached to your mouth like a little tube. They remain in a *ring, sealed* to your mouth so your mouth doesn't have to create the pressure with your lips wrapped over your teeth. No more worn-out inside lips. And your jaw doesn't get tired trying maintain pressure. No more TMJ. Your hand attached to your mouth has elongated the area of possible stimulation for him, from the three to four inches of your mouth to six to eight inches with your hand. Also, your thumb and finger create the pressure and allow you to relax your mouth more, buffered by your lips. This lets you be in control of the speed and strength with which he enters your mouth and also creates further pressure for him.

The request for deep-throating is often a result of the visual cues from the adult film world, which is notorious for its high degree of fabrication. In other words, deep-throating is nearly impossible for most women. If you are controlling the pace and the placement in which his penis enters your mouth, and using the Ring, there's very little chance of your gagging. You can decide how far that penis goes, and once you've reached your maximum level of comfort, you then simply pull it back out. As his penis begins to feel more comfortable in your mouth, you will gradually be able to take in more of it, should that be what you desire.

> ### SECRET FROM LOU'S ARCHIVES
>
> *Men have said it is the combination of three things that absolutely makes for entering a woman vaginally during sex: the combination of heat, pressure, and moisture. Keep this in mind when giving oral sex: Your mouth creates the moisture and your hand in the ring shape, sealed to your mouth can create a lot more sensation than another area of your body. Use that to your advantage.*

If you remember nothing else about performing oral sex on a man, let it be this: In order for it to be done effectively, *you* must be in charge. This is something you do for *him,* not something he does for himself *through* you.

MOUTH MAGIC

There are four main components that combine to create great oral sex. Like dancing, sometimes you put all the steps together in one move and other times you slow down the pace, but more than likely you are constantly varying your moves to the beat and according to how you feel at the moment.

It won't take long to discover that the secret to giving great oral sex is to find your "rhythm," and that rhythm, as in dancing, can and will change with each partner, depending on his specific likes and dislikes. What will ensure your success with every encounter is to remember the four different motions you use whenever performing oral sex. When and how you use them will depend on your rhythm, but the motions themselves are always the same. And FYI, the more manual you do on him the less time the oral is likely to take.

> You *seal* your hand to your mouth in the *ring* shape. Or, if you want just use your mouth but it will be more tiring.

> Your mouth (with teeth covered) is moving up and down his shaft to increase length of the stimulation area for him.

> Your tongue is always moving in a back-and-forth or circular motion across the frenulum area, which is the V-shaped notch at the back of the head of the penis. This allows him to feel the more textured tastebud surface throughout the experience.

> Your free hand is stimulating another part of his body, such as the nipples, inner thighs, perineal area, or anus, in order to broaden the area of sensual pleasure.

As long as you don't forget these four movements, your oral sex experiences are always going to be pleasurable for both of you. And though I've said this before, I think it bears repeating once again. The joy you derive out of pleasing him is worth its weight in gold—of that there is no doubt. But knowing you alone possess the ability to deliver it is likely to do more to reflect your power as a woman than anything you can even imagine. So don't overlook the pleasure you are capable of giving your lover. For many men, oral sex is one of their most satisfying experiences.

On the subject of swallowing, or allowing him to come in your mouth: your mouth, your choice; but I will say that "well-balanced nice-guy men" have said they like it because it makes them feel one of the most masculine parts of them has been accepted. Should you choose to do so, you can heighten the sensation he feels when ejaculating, either in or not in your mouth, by pulsing your now still hands wrapped around his shaft in time with the ejaculations.

If you put the steps together, it should look like this:

1. Use your hands to form the Ring and Seal. Remember your hand stays *attached* at all times to your mouth.

2. Move your mouth up and down the length of his shaft, while maintaining a comfortable level of suction. You won't have to create much suction as your Ring can create the sensation of suction when you do the upward stroke. At the same time, your *sealed* hand, the one attached to your mouth, is doing a *twisting motion* while you are going up and down his shaft.

3. Keep your tongue in constant motion, across the frenulum, and you can use either the tastebud surface or the smooth underside to create sensation.

4. Don't forget to mind the stepchildren. Named so by a seminar attendee because "they belong to someone else and they often get ignored," invariably his testicles like to be held,

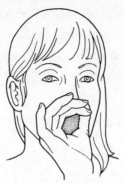

Forming the Seal and the Ring

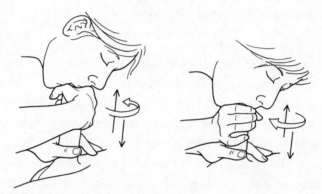

Step 2: Moving up and down the shaft . . . while twisting

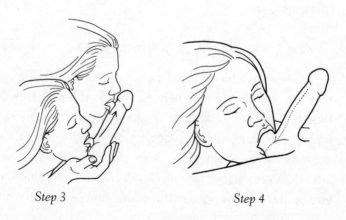

Step 3   *Step 4*

fondled, and warmed in your hands or mouth, so move occasionally to lick the scrotum and testicles. Worried about hair? Gently stroke the area beforehand to remove any loose little hairs. Ask him to hold your hand on them in the way he prefers.

5. Let your free hand roam the rest of his body.

6. Look him in the eye. Consider asking him to watch you.

Prostate and Anal Orgasms

Analogous to a woman's G-spot, the prostate as you know by now can be stimulated either externally or internally, and some men also enjoy being stimulated externally on the anus as well. The prostate can be stimulated by use of fingers (she should definitely use a lubricant without nonoxynol-9, which can be irritating) or with a toy, such as a dildo or butt plug, depending on how "full" a man likes to feel when penetrated. In any of these cases, it's also necessary to use lubricant so that no tissue irritation occurs. Remember, this isn't a self-lubricating area.

ROSE PETALS (AKA ANILINGUS)

For women who are comfortable with anilingus, some men who are sensitive to anal play may enjoy this technique. For this the woman will use her tongue like a soft sculpting tool on his anus. And again, I suggest incorporating other complimentary moves at the same time. A favorite among seminar attendees is to be performing Rose Petals on his behind while giving him a hand job at the same time—the intensity of

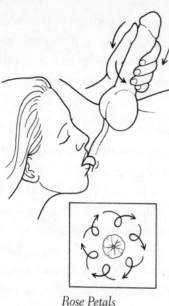

the sensation can make his orgasm sensational!

The best position for anilingus is to have your man on all fours, facing away from you or lying on his back with his hips on a pillow. This support allows a more tilted pelvis, which makes his anal area more available to you. More than one woman has asked, "How do I get him on all fours?" My suggestion: Simply ask him to get in that position. Chances are he'll get there in a blink.

Rose Petals

With him facing away from you, use a strong stroking motion with your tongue. Imagine you are creating the sepals (the small green leaves at the bottom of a rose) and circle the rim of his anus (this is known as rimming). The off-the-charts move is to incorporate hand stimulation while your hot, moist mouth is on his anus. This can be accomplished in one of two ways: (1) reach your hand around his thigh and use a gentle pulling stroke toward the head of his penis. Make sure to use a warm, well-lubricated hand; (2) reach between his legs and, using one hand on his penis, do a smooth, forward, stroking, gentle twisting motion toward his shoulders.

HISTORICAL AND HYSTERICAL FACTS	Anal intercourse is the most popular sexual practice depicted in pre-Columbian art.

Anal play definitely can add a new dimension to your sexual repertoire, but don't feel pressure to add it if you are uncomfortable. Talk with each other and see if you are both interested in experimenting in this perfectly natural way.

Fantasy Orgasm

In my eight years of doing seminars, I have only met one man who is capable of orgasming without any physical stimulation at all. He says it is all about his willpower and mental control. Now, whether one can climax with fantasy alone or fantasy plus some stimulation, this is an area that has as much variation as people have imagination. Often fantasies have their roots in youthful experiences—be it the cool plastic apron of your mother or nanny who held you after the bath that lead to your enjoyment of latex, or the excitement you felt when you saw your next-door neighbor silhouetted through her bedroom window. Then there are fantasies that require others' participation. Often masturbation fantasies are best left for solo enjoyment, as the reality (or translation) never seems to match the mental experience.

Fantasy has a strange sexual power. There are ways to enhance your sexual experience through certain sources, such as erotic stories, magazines, videos, sharing fantasies with your partner, or pure imagination. This is all a matter of taste and knowing what turns you both on. I generally caution against using erotic sources if one of you is uncomfortable.

Nipple / Breast Orgasm

I know of only one man who is able to come based on the stimulation of his nipples. But I figure if there is one man, there are others. The man I spoke with said that if a woman merely licks, sucks, and nibbles on his nipples the right way he is sent into the stratosphere! "It is illegal how good this feels," he told me. So do not overlook that a good number of men get turned on by gentle biting, nibbling, or licking on this erogenous zone. You can stimulate his nipples with your tongue, teeth, hands, and fingers, or with toys such as nipple clips and suction cups. These are designed for the area and come in vibrating versions as well. Of course, there are other men, as there are women, who don't like this at all. As always, it's best to communicate with your partner.

Toys

As you no doubt know by now, toys are not just for children! I'm a big proponent of adding toys into a couple's sexual repertoire because they add fun, spice, and variety.

Men who like anal play enjoy both butt plugs and anal beads. Those who like to increase the intensity of their erection often play with cock rings. There are a number of toys that I describe in chapter 8, where I talk about enhancing your sexual experience. If you're interested, you might want to jump ahead now.

Sex for One

Although men are generally more comfortable than women with the notion and practice of masturbation, there still exist shameful or secretive associations with a man's desire, need, or preference to pleasure himself. Some men report that even though they have wonderful sex lives with their partners, they still like to "do themselves." Their reasons vary: some say they like the autonomy and not having to worry about anyone else's feelings; others say "it's like an urge . . . and I want to do it quickly."

In my experience with women and men in my seminars, one of the best (most effective) ways that men and women can have their easiest and best orgasm is from masturbating, which is often the way they first learned to orgasm. That nerve response pathway is already set and your body knows what to expect. So one of the simpler ways to show or direct your partner as to how you like to be touched or stimulated is to show her what you do. Now, I'm sure some of you may not be comfortable with the concept of masturbating. Please know that I maintain that we should never have to do anything we don't want to. These are our bodies, and our choices.

However, if you are comfortable with or curious about how masturbation techniques can lead to better self-knowledge and ultimately to a stronger, more intense, or more pleasurable orgasm, then without further ado, help yourself.

Dr. Bernie Zilbergeld points out in his book *The New Male Sexuality* three very positive reasons for masturbation:

> ➤ Self-pleasuring is an excellent way to learn how you like to be touched and stimulated, not only on your genitals, but elsewhere as well. This information can then be given to your partner, thus enhancing your sex life together.

> ➤ Even if you're committed to partner sex as the best way of satisfying your erotic needs, there may be times when you don't have a partner or the partner you do have isn't available because of illness, fatigue, or

something else. Why deny yourself sexual pleasure at such times?

➤ Masturbating can also help to overcome sexual problems such as erection difficulties and rapid or premature ejaculation. (I go into this in more detail in chapter 7.)

Dr. Zilbergeld also points out that the only way masturbation might be bad is when a man regularly uses it as a substitute for sex with his partner. Obviously, this would not be good for his relationship and I'm sure the woman would feel extraneous or not important.

Here are some techniques for increasing your pleasure while masturbating:

➤ Using a silk scarf, cup your testicles as you touch yourself. This will give you new and different tactile sensations, and can heighten your sensitivity to touch.

➤ If she's comfortable, invite your partner to partake by having her hold your testicles or shaft and having her nestle in close to you as you touch yourself.

➤ Use a lubricant that helps to maintain a smooth flow of motion when you are pleasuring yourself.

Men, like women, should feel comfortable exploring their own range of orgasmic pleasure. The techniques and types described in this chapter are meant to prompt interest and curiosity, not pressure you into anything that may feel uncomfortable. However, we all know our own "short cuts" to orgasm, so trying some alternatives may lead to wider horizons. By all means, enjoy yourselves!

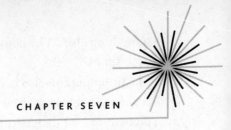

CHAPTER SEVEN

Medical Concerns That Impact Sexuality

"Maintaining your sexual health
is a lifelong process."
—Dr. Richard Milsten

Take Care of That Body

For all of us when our bodies are operating well, everything in our lives operates well, including our sex life. Like a finely tuned motor, we hum. However, if just one cylinder is misfiring, we are out of sorts and can't complete the course. How fabulous that as human beings we have so many different facets by which we can experience sex—mentally, physically, and spiritually! However, there are also many different ways that the sexual flow can be interrupted or derailed.

The point of this chapter is to expand your knowledge of medical issues that impact your ability to have the orgasm you desire. For women, this may be as simple as understanding the connection between your menstrual cycle (ovulation cycle) and your libido (you might find that sometimes you are more sensitive genitally and more interested in sex). Women who may have at one time or another experienced periods of low desire may find out the reasons behind the trouble connected to their lust factor. And women who are anorgasmic (unable to have an orgasm) will learn the likely causes and possible solutions. There are women for whom not having an orgasm is not an issue; and as with all things in life, it isn't an issue until you say it is. Some physical concerns that impact women's sexuality include vaginal dryness, vaginal tightness, cramping or pain, and bacterial or viral infections that can lead to more serious sexual problems, including PIDs (pelvic inflammatory diseases) and endometriosis.

Sore joints, hips, backs, knees, and fingers impact all of us—not just women; these joint problems are further aggravated by arthritis, which of course cuts across gender lines. As a seventy-three-year-old woman told me, "I could do whatever I wanted at forty, that changed slightly at fifty, and again at sixty. Now at seventy-three, there are some things I'd love to try again, but I just can't bend that way anymore. My knees and hips can't take it. I have to be creative."

HISTORICAL AND HYSTERICAL FACTS	In New Ireland, a husband and wife did not have intercourse while their pig was pregnant, and did not indulge until one month after it gave birth.

For men, the many medical and physical issues that affect sexuality revolve around the penis, most especially with a fear of premature ejaculation and impotence or the inability to attain an erection firm enough for penetration. I also address other medical conditions that impact sexual functioning.

As you probably know, many of the medications for such conditions as high blood pressure, diabetes, depression or anxiety, and heart disease do impact both desire (i.e., libido) and full sexual physiological functioning. (There is a chart of many of the medications impacting sexual functioning at the end of this chapter.) The first step to addressing issues of medications is to become aware; the second is to consult your physician and see if there are any alternative medications that have fewer or no negative side effects to sexual functioning. Also, I will present some suggestions that may help "skirt" the problems, so to speak. Medical concerns are real, but most are treatable if you take the time to address them thoroughly. You should take your sexual health seriously, and the first step is learning what might affect you—either now or in the future.

| HISTORICAL AND HYSTERICAL FACTS | I am in agreement with Dr. Gloria Brame who writes, "What if all this 'dysfunction' is not so much a lack of interest in sex, but a lack of interest in the type of sex that society considers normal?" |

Let's Ban the "Dys" of Sexual Functioning

One of my real pet peeves when it comes to dealing with sexual functioning is how quick the media and the medical establishment are to jump to conclusions and label a problem or difficulty with orgasm as a "dysfunction." The language alone is enough to deter women and men from seeking help, asking questions, and becoming creative in their search for solutions.

I think we already have established that what we tend to call "normal" isn't all that broad or accurate—especially in terms of sexuality. To tell people they have a *dys*function sets people back, increasing their hesitancy to speak up about their problems.

In many situations, though, there may be physiological causes to sexual problems, and there are often psychological cures. For instance, although it's true that as women age and leave the realm of their childbearing years (mid-forties), their bodies are undergoing tremendous hormonal changes. But how is this shifting around in hormones different from what was happening during puberty? Pregnancy? Your monthly cycle? My point is that women, especially those who are familiar with their bodies' cycles and fluxes, are used to hormonal changes. When, as they approach and pass through menopause, they find themselves a bit drier, it does not mean they are automatically experiencing a decrease in desire. They simply need to use a lubricant to help things along. In fact, many women over forty with whom I've worked say the opposite: Now that they are more comfortable with themselves, their bodies, and, if they are in a relationship, with their partners, they are more comfortable wanting and asking for sexual satisfaction.

SECRET FROM LOU'S ARCHIVES

Attention men! Menopause does not signal an end to women's sexual interest and satisfaction.

The typical source of information about hormonal changes is women who are going through the same thing. So it makes sense that men wouldn't have a lot of information in this area. We are now seeing the first generation of women who are publicly redefining female sexuality postmenopausally.

The same case can be made for men. Young men are notorious for their ability to have sex more than once a day; before they hit their thirties, it's as if their testosterone is on overdrive, pushing them in some kind of instinctual frenzy to release their sperm. Once in their thirties, however, they naturally slow down, and by the time men are in their fifties and sixties, they are on a much more even keel—their desire more balanced with their instincts. This is a natural, universal process—not a sign of dysfunction.

The following list about the normal changes in sexual function with aging for men is from Milsten and Slowinski's book *The Sexual Male*:

1. It takes longer to achieve an erection.
2. The duration of ejaculation decreases from between four and eight seconds to approximately three seconds.
3. The volume of ejaculate is reduced from approximately one teaspoon to less than half that amount.
4. The force with which the semen is expelled decreases so that it is projected from the end of the penis a distance of only two to twelve inches instead of twelve to twenty-four inches.
5. The time from erection to ejaculation may increase.
6. Following ejaculation, the penis becomes softer much more rapidly.
7. The time before the next erection can be achieved is prolonged.
8. The weight of the testicles decreases.

9. The tactile sensitivity of the penis is decreased.
10. The intensity of the orgasm may decrease.
11. The angle of the erection may decrease.

So as you can see, in these normal changes there is nothing about impotence. As Slowinski and Milsten further comment, "Erectile ability is in fact associated with a male's general health status."

I believe that the more men and women accept their bodies, their age, and their own desire level, the more comfortable they will be with their sexuality in general. Further, the more comfortable they are, the more likely they will be to explore and discover the absolute heights to their own pleasure. It goes without saying (and I know I've said this earlier in the book) that seeking and finding one's absolute pleasure are an individual thing. There are no bar codes, no polls, no statistics or definitions of pleasure that should define *your* orgasm. If you are satisfied with your orgasm, then that is what is best for you. Full stop!

SECRET FROM LOU'S ARCHIVES

The truth is that erectile insufficiency is not caused by aging. It is a phenomenon that occurs with the onset of other illnesses, and since the likelihood of illness increases with age, so does impotence. As males grow older, certain alterations in sexual functioning do occur.

Do You Have Low Desire?

My problem with the phrase "low desire" is its ubiquitous nature. It seems that every publication you pick up—whether it is a men's or women's magazine—there's an article stressing how Americans, especially women, "suffer" from low sexual desire. In a recent *O* (Oprah's magazine), the editors claimed that over 25 million women have experienced low sexual desire. Now, if someone asked you whether you had low or high desire, how would you answer? I would guess that most of us have high desire some of the time and low desire at other times. When you're in a new relationship, don't you experience a rush of desire? Don't you feel more passionate? Once a relationship has a few years on it, wouldn't you agree that it's natural that the lust factor can wane? What about the stresses of work, family, and personal issues? Don't you believe that the day-to-day demands of life in general take their toll on our feeling sexually open and wanting?

It is my observation that the pharmaceutical industry is looking for a new cash cow and that cash cow would be a drug to treat the "sexual dysfunctions" they have "discovered." The medical establishment, spearheaded by the pharmaceutical industry, has begun to define low desire as a disease and one that can only be treated by prescription drugs. Now, I am not arguing the merits of Viagra, but I am questioning the drug companies' underlying motivation and definition of low desire. Low desire is an experience many women and men have that is the result of more than one factor. It's my conviction that as we know more about our own bodies, and connect our bodies to what is happening in the rest of our lives, we will begin to unravel the reasons why we may have become disconnected from our libidos. After all, why do we need drugs to get in touch with what is the most natural thing about us, our sexuality?

And while I don't deny that low desire exists, I regret that doctors, counselors, other women, men, and the media in general alarm people about this. Low desire is not a fact of life, nor is it an unchangeable medical condition. Rather, low desire is often transient, often subjective, and often in reaction to many stresses in our lives, including fatigue and everyday pressures of home, family, and work. I prefer to address low desire less as a problem and more as an experience, one that needs to be recognized and acknowledged, certainly, but one that also needs to be understood in order to deal with it.

That said, there are cases where low desire can be directly linked to physiological causes, such as men or women experiencing hormonal imbalances or going through serious illnesses. And it makes sense because stress is one of the biggest interrupters of sexuality, and when we are emotionally or physically stressed, our sexuality usually takes a holiday.

Let's first take a look at the physiological issues that impact women's and men's sexual health.

The Women: From Preorgasmia to Nirvana

I have gathered here the major medical conditions affecting or impacting sexual functioning in women. This is by no means complete, but it will direct you to the most common and most serious. If any of these situations applies to you—either in whole or in part—I recommend you consult with your physician as soon as possible.

Preorgasmia (aka Anorgasmia)

The media and popular polls have thrown around a lot of numbers about how many women do or don't experience orgasms. A recent Chicago study published in the *Journal of the American Medical Association* (*JAMA*) stated that 22–28 percent of women in different age categories were unable to achieve orgasm during intercourse. If this is you and you are interested, I want you to know that having an orgasm is not only possible, it's probable. This may not be true in all situations, but rather in those that will work for you. As I noted in chapter 1, according to Kate White, editor in chief of *Cosmopolitan* magazine, her readers' most common question is "How do I have an orgasm during intercourse?" The pressure for women to have an orgasm from male-superior sex has done both sexes a huge disservice. Quite simply this position and action are not the most efficient way for women to come. Perhaps this works for porn stars in which the so-called plot is generally directed at stimulating a man's masturbatory fantasy—not giving real women and men a realistic picture of a woman having an orgasm.

Believe me. I've spoken with countless women who went from believing they would never, ever have an orgasm to being able to orgasm easily. Other women learned with practice and getting to know their bodies' preferences, which includes being able to do so whenever they wished. Having an orgasm can be a straightforward procedure: it's a matter of getting to know your body, relaxing into your body, and learning how and what stimulates you. If you have personal or emotional issues that seem to interfere with your sexual pleasure, then it's best to work on these at the same time that you're trying to learn how to orgasm. I am not a therapist or a psychologist, so I would recommend seeking a professional with whom to consult.

A number of women in private session have told me in

confidence that they are not at all sure whether they have ever had an orgasm. I believe them. If you don't know what you're looking for, you may not recognize it. One woman told me that she had tried to orgasm with a vibrator but it didn't work. It turns out that she was using it too intensely on her clitoris and numbing herself. I asked if she was holding her breath while masturbating, and she said yes, that it helped her concentrate. The solution was simple: She shifted the vibrator's focus to her outer labia and used a short up-and-down stroke along the clitoral ridge, concentrating on deep, even, slow breaths. Later she told me, "Oh, my God. It is all about the breathing. Why did no one ever tell me that? And that on-the-side thing—man, I can do this again and again and not get numb!" Needless to say she was both relieved and filled with wonderful pleasure at discovering she could indeed orgasm.

Many therapists will recommend that a woman learn to masturbate in order to know what she likes, and I've provided these techniques in chapter 5. However, if you aren't comfortable with that or have never done it before, the best starting point is getting more comfortable with your own body. This lack of familiarity is often the biggest barrier. Getting to know yourself may be as simple as taking the time to look at yourself nude in a mirror or by touching yourself and paying attention to how that part of your body feels when touched. We human beings are rather crazy in this department. Why is it okay for a woman to have her partner touch her "down there," but not herself? It's not as if her body doesn't belong to her. Au contraire!

The following are a few tried-and-true techniques others have used to expand their own awareness and learn new ways to stimulate themselves. All women don't do all things. Like our taste in clothes, it is very individualistic.

> Start by learning what sensations work—soft, rough, cool, warm, etc.
> Then, over a period of days or weeks, move to more direct genital stimulation, using either your hand, fingers, water jets from a showerhead or Jacuzzi, or using a dildo or vibrator. Think of this as seducing yourself, because in all actuality that is what you are doing.

Vaginismus

A tightening of the entry of the vagina (the first third of the vaginal canal) can make intercourse painful, if not impossible. Deep pelvic pain may inhibit sexual responsiveness either from disease or inflammation in the uterus or ovaries, awkward positions, or lack of sufficient arousal during sex. Vaginismus is an involuntary contraction of these muscles and may be the result of the woman's body trying to prevent an action (i.e., it's a warning signal). There are also psychological components that play a role here, especially if the original problem can be traced to a traumatic gynecological exam, poor body image, or fear and anxiety about anything penetrating the vagina. Women who suffer from vulvar vestibulitis (see page 159) can experience vaginismus as a secondary result.

Reduced Vaginal Lubrication

Extraordinary or excessive vaginal dryness can result from nursing, recent delivery, antihistamines or other medications, and a general, overall lack of hydration. Dryness can also be a response to shifting hormone levels during menopause, as well as the thinning of the vaginal mucosal tissue. In extreme cases, some women have even experienced painful dry cracks in the vaginal mucosa (or lining). The solution for this condition is quite simple: water-based lubricants that are safe when introduced vaginally. (See more on lubricants in chapter 8.)

Endometriosis

This condition is a result of the endometrial tissue (from the endometrium, the lining of the uterus) shed monthly during a woman's period becoming implanted on the other internal organs, such as the fallopian tubes or ovaries. Endometriosis can be extremely painful or completely asymptomatic. Women usually experience pain during ovulation and increased hormonal levels.

Vulvodynia (aka Vulvar Vestibulitis)

This is an old problem with a new name, point out Slowinski and Milsten. Other terms cited in the medical literature refer to this condition as "burning vulva syndrome." Vulvodynia is a feeling of vaginal burning that some women experience before, during, or after and even apart from any sexual activity. Many of these women come to their doctors with a complaint of vaginismus and localized pain near the vaginal entrance. They describe it as a "hot spot" that when touched can cause sharp pain ("like a paper cut"). There may also be more than one point of painful sensitivity. The existence and diagnosis of vulvodynia have caused gynecologists and women patients much confusion and frustration for years.

Urinary Tract Infections

Urinary Tract Infections (UTI) are very common among women of all ages and can be caused by many factors, including having sex, changes in soaps used genitally, and/or douching. Although UTIs are highly treatable with either an antibiotic or a more organic, homeopathic remedy (they work—believe me!), they can make sex painful or undesirable. The common symptoms of UTIs are pain and burning during urination and sexual intercourse.

Yeast Infections

A yeast infection in women does not necessarily impact sexual functioning, but they make women uncomfortable "down there," inhibiting their desire for sex. The common symptom of a *yeast infection* is heavier than normal discharge of the kind that is thick and sticky and it is sometimes accompanied by a stronger smell, as well as an itching, burning sensation. There are good over-the-counter medications that treat yeast infections quickly without any harmful side effects; your doctor can also prescribe a stronger remedy in a higher dosage, but be sure you are indeed treating a yeast infection and not something else, such as bacterial vaginosis.

Bladder Infections

Bladder infections are usually accompanied by a frequent need to urinate, and/or a burning sensation when you urinate. A home remedy that works for many women is drinking a lot of cranberry juice. The blend of high acids apparently makes it impossible for one strain of the bacteria that causes the infection to adhere to the bladder wall. Cranberry juice works for some but not all organisms causing an infection. So if the symptoms persist, you should consult your physician for more medical advice and treatment.

Bacterial Vaginosis (BV)

This very common infection is what often causes that strong "fishy" smell some women have noticed in their vaginal secretions. Most women are not even aware that they have BV until they notice the smell, and the smell is often only noticed after a woman has unprotected sex with a man who ejaculates inside of her. In this case, when her vaginal secretions come in contact with semen, an amine group (a nitrogen-containing organic compound) is released and the fishy smell is detected. This is easily diagnosed and treated with antibacterial medications. If left untreated, BV may cause complications, including abnormal pap smears and increased risk of pelvic inflammatory disease (PID), and in pregnancy it has been associated with premature birth and low-birth-weight infants. Although BV in and of itself does not inhibit desire, it can be a turnoff because of the strong odor often accompanying it.

SECRET FROM LOU'S ARCHIVES

Dr. Jules Black, OB/GYN, states that the most common cause of UTIs, yeast infections, and vaginosis is deficient hygiene, caused by wiping forward after defecation and urination, bringing naturally occurring organisms from the bowel to where they don't belong, the vagina and urethra. Women must use a positive wipe from front to back.

The Men

When men are bothered by problems affecting their genitals, they often don't have the built-in "lets talk about it" response that women have. Yet when this sensitive area of a man's anatomy is having problems, he does want to deal with it quickly. As one man told me, "I do not want Johnny having problems. When he has something wrong, I have something wrong."

If it is pain or an infection, invariably men head to the doctor. There is no stigma attached to any of the possible conditions. Unlike women, men rarely have a problem with telling a doctor they had sex and think they may have "caught something." Symptoms that will bring a man in for an exam can be a complaint of a burning sensation when they ejaculate or pain in the testicles or around the anal opening at or shortly after ejaculation. What I've gathered below is the most current information about sexual health considerations.

There are many health conditions that can negatively impact sexual functioning in men. Here is a list of those to be aware of:

Addison's disease (adrenal insufficiency)
Alcoholism
Anemia (severe)
Anorexia nervosa
Chronic active hepatitis
Chronic kidney failure
Cirrhosis
Congestive heart failure
Cushing's syndrome

Depression

Drug addiction

Drug ingestion: antiandrogens, antihypertensives, digoxin, estrogen, tranquilizers

Excessive prolactin secretion (drug or tumor induced)

Feminizing tumors

Hemochromatosis

Hypothyroidism

Kallmann's syndrome

Klinefelter's syndrome

Male climacteric (with testosterone deficiency)

Multiple sclerosis

Myotonic dystrophy

Nutritional deficiencies

Parkinson's disease

Pituitary insufficiency

Pituitary tumors

Testosterone deficiency

Tuberculosis

(Source: Masters, W. H., V. E. Johnson, and R. C. Kolodny, *Heterosexuality*, 1994, p. 86)

If you or your partner suffers from one or more of these conditions, know first that your sexuality may be affected. You should consult with a physician to see about necessary treatment.

The following conditions more directly relate to the genitals and therefore impact sexual functioning more immediately.

Prostatitis

Prostatitis is an inflammation of the prostate gland caused by a bacterial infection. This is often accompanied by fever and back pains, a general overall feeling of being ill, and a searing sensation that burns through the penis and urinary tract. An aggressive use of antibiotics can treat the infection.

Chronic Prostatitis

This somewhat more rare but more serious condition is caused by a chronic infection to the prostate gland that ends up affecting the seminal vesicles as well. When both these glands are chronically swollen, they press on surrounding nerves and thereby short-circuit during urination and sexual arousal. One researcher said it's like angina, in the characteristic way it spreads. There is no certain cause for this infection; boys who have never had sex can suffer from it as much as a sexually active adult man.

Impotence or Penile Erectile Dysfunction

Getting an erection is the essence of many men's sexuality, and therefore an inability to become erect or maintain an erection for a desired length of time can be an enormously burdensome experience for most men. Although impotence can strike men at any age—including teenagers—it is often associated with men over age fifty-five. Here are some numbers:

- ➤ At age fifty-five, 8 percent of healthy men suffer from it.
- ➤ At age sixty-five, 25 percent of men.
- ➤ At seventy-five, 55 percent.
- ➤ At eighty, as many as 75 percent of men experience. the frustration of impotence.

According to Dr. Irwin Goldstein, there are three main physiological reasons men suffer from erectile dysfunction:

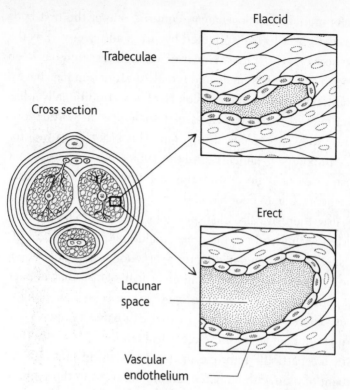

Flaccid

Trabeculae

Cross section

Erect

Lacunar
space

Vascular
endothelium

Blood Flow to Flaccid and Erect Penis

(1) failure to initiate; (2) failure to fill; and (3) failure to store. Failure to initiate is a fancy way of describing what happens when important nerves in the penis fail to function correctly in response to sexual stimulation, which may be caused by low hormone levels. Failure to fill means just that—not enough arterial high-pressure blood gets to the penis to expand the penile tissue. Failure to store indicates that the erection-storage mechanism is unable to expand to its maximum against the tunica, or fibrous coat to maintain the blood in the penile tissue.

As many psychologists can confirm, one of the first body organs to be adversely affected by stress and overwork is the one between the thighs. However, enough research has been done to suggest that male and female dysfunction may have a common molecular and physiological link. Traditionally it has been viewed that most cases of female sexual dysfunctions were purely psychological in origin. This was true as well for male impotence—at least until the 1980s. Now we know that most cases of male dysfunction are physiological in cause, specifically due to poor blood flow.

Also, there are also clear physiological links to men's difficulties getting and staying erect, including most physical illnesses. As mentioned in chapter 3, erection is dependent on a man's nervous system sending electrical signals that impact the penis and cause blood to engorge the vessels, making it erect. There are many illnesses that can cause temporary or permanent damage to these electrical circuits. Men with diabetes are particularly prone to this problem; in fact, 50–70 percent of men with diabetes (2.5 million men in the United States) suffer from impotence. This is partly because of damage to nerves, but it's also due in part to disturbances in their metabolism.

A prolapsed disk, any operation to pelvic organs, including surgery for hernias, and multiple sclerosis can also cause erection problems. Aging, as we see above, is a natural, overall factor affecting erectile functioning, and as I point out below in the section on hormones, hormonal changes weigh heavily here.

According to Taoist physician Dr. Mantak Chia, erection trouble is caused not only by physiological and psychological problems, but also by an energetic problem, specifically, weak sexual energy. Difficulty in getting or maintaining an erection is understood as resulting from a man's physical and sexual exhaustion. The general Taoist approach to sex emphasizes energy currents.

It should make plain sense that if you are doing something that is going to impact your circulatory system either positively (i.e., working out) or negatively (i.e., smoking and drinking), your sexual functioning will be affected. Why? Because blood and good circulation are the two things that power orgasms. You smoke? That, gentlemen, is one of the quicker ways to reduce penile functioning. The majority of blood vessels in the penis are tiny, and the tinier they are, the faster blood impairment will weaken an area. There was a great billboard advertisement with several men standing around in tuxedos smoking. A pretty woman walks by and all their cigarettes drooped over like wilted flowers. The message was clear: If you smoke, you reduce your most masculine function. As Drs. Milsten and Slowinski point out, "The evidence is overwhelming that the use of tobacco causes impairment of blood flow not only to the heart but also to the penis. Recent data suggests these changes may not be reversible, so it is important to avoid damage in the first place."

This is also true of significant alcohol consumption. Dr. Irwin Goldstein says in his book *The Potent Male* that "heavy drinking of alcohol, over time, may destroy the ability of a man to make love. Too much alcohol may reduce the production of the testosterone in the testicles. Since heavy drinking also impairs liver function, and the liver is responsible for metabolizing hormones, the reduced amount of hormones may not be enough for proper penile functioning. Heavy drinking may also damage a man's nervous system, which is vital to sexual functioning. . . . Prolonged use of cocaine and marijuana also result in erection problems." Frankly, I would think these warnings about using any kind of drug—legal or otherwise—would convince men to be careful and be moderate in their behavior. Lifestyle changes aren't necessarily easy, but if potency and sexual health is important to you, you may find the motivation.

For men, I recommend ways of learning how to stimulate and maintain stimulation in order to stay erect longer (if that's your wish) and to better control ejaculation. I describe and discuss these in chapters 8 and 9, when I address ways to enhance orgasms (through better erection and ejaculatory control) and Eastern Taoist and Tantric techniques that also aid in sexual control and health.

Rapid Ejaculation (aka Lack of Ejaculation Control)

Rapid ejaculation occurs when a man ejaculates either before entering the vagina or shortly thereafter, in either case, before he wants to. Traditional teaching has been that psychological issues are at the root of this problem, yet another school of thought is that it is just another of many physical differences between men. The American Psychiatric Association defines rapid, aka premature, ejaculation as the "persistent or recurrent ejaculation with minimal sexual stimulation before, during or shortly after penetration and before the person wishes it." Despite these slightly different definitions, rapid ejaculation remains a frustrating circumstance for both the men and the women involved. As sexologist Helen Kaplan states, "It simply isn't known how long the average male takes to ejaculate. Given the naturally competitive nature of men, if an actually well-adjusted man reads he should take X amount of time and he takes Y, he may start to feel inadequate, even though his partner is satisfied." That aside, women do get frustrated. One woman told me, "He was the best guy, but he would come as soon as he was inside me and I needed more. He's now married to a great woman and said the timing that was a problem for us is the ticket for the two of them."

The other side of the coin is delayed ejaculation, which can be as difficult to deal with. The woman can get very sore vaginally or orally, and still he is unable to orgasm. In this kind of situation, a woman can feel that no matter what she does, she isn't doing "something" right.

According to some experts, as high as 40 percent of men have at some time had problems with ejaculation. Especially when a man is young and virile, premature ejaculation can cause anxiety and noticeably affect his enjoyment of the climax (as well as that of his partner).

Since for many men an erection and the ability to control ejaculation is associated with feelings of strength, control, and power, they often experience tremendous feelings of inadequacy when premature ejaculation happens. As men age, and they expect some of their physical functioning to wane, they take it less to heart.

There are three different approaches to the treatment of premature ejaculation. The first approach utilizes counseling as a way to deal with and address the psychological dimensions of the behavior. Let's be honest: If a man feels that the part of his anatomy that he believes most identifies him as a man is out of his control, he will definitely have some psychological issues.

The second approach is behavior modification. A popular method is the "stop-start" technique, which boils down to exercises a man can learn to do to control ejaculation—either with a partner or solo. The Kegel exercises discussed in chapter 8 are an example of this approach.

The third approach is the recent use of pharmacological drugs. Most of these drugs were found to work on premature ejaculation secondarily. For example, Prozac, which is used for depression, delays ejaculation. The same occurs with the drug Anafranil, normally used for obsessive-compulsive behavior.

For any man (or couple) who is bothered by premature ejaculation, I would consider all three approaches to see what is most suitable for you.

Our Hormonal Soup and Its Sexual Ingredients

Hormones are those elusive, fascinating body chemicals that make women and men sexual beings. They are powerful and have a tremendous effect on our bodies and minds. Therefore, when hormone levels in the body are unbalanced, the body will respond, and often negatively, especially in terms of sexual functioning. The main hormones that affect men's and women's sexuality are estrogen, testosterone, and progesterone. I provide below a summary of the importance of these hormones to sexual functioning, and indicate what happens sexually when hormones are unbalanced. This is not a complete discussion of hormonal effects throughout the body, but use this information as a guideline to ask yourself if you or your partner might not be connecting sexually due to a hormonal imbalance. Much of this information on hormones comes from a trusted medical source—Dr. Lana Holstein, who discusses how hormones affect sex in her book, *How to Have Magnificent Sex*. If you think or suspect that one or more of these situations applies to you, you will need to contact your physician.

Estrogen—The Key to Women's Vitality

Estrogen is vital to women's proper sexual functioning. There are three major estrogens in the body: estrone, estriol, and estradiol. Estradiol is the most potent of the three. Women's major source of estradiol is the follicle, or egg sac, of the ovary. When these follicles are depleted at menopause, or when the ovaries are removed surgically or their function destroyed by chemotherapy or radiation, women often experience a tremendous loss of sexual desire and other changes to their sexual functioning. To replace this important hormone, women can use a vaginal lubricant, as well as estrogen vaginal creams, oral supplements, or skin patches. A new form of replacement estrogen is a silicone ring, the Estring™, which resembles a diaphragm and releases a small amount of estrogen daily. The ring contains the equivalent of two days' worth of an oral dosage that is then very gradually released over three months. This ring can even stay in place in the vagina during intercourse and releases estrogen only to the local tissue, avoiding the systemic blood levels of estrogen. Many women who are leery of taking estrogen or who have medical constraints find the ring a great alternative to messy vaginal estrogen creams.

Although there is still great confusion and debate about whether or not to take estrogen, most women understand that there are both benefits and risks to hormone replacement therapy. It is a very individual choice and one that every woman should discuss with her physician and other trusted people in her life. There is an increasing variety of preparations now available, so that each woman can decide whether or not to use a patch, pill, or cream, or nothing at all. We are receiving new data about estrogen on a daily basis, so until we (and the scientific and medical communities) have complete knowledge of the pros and cons of hormone replacement therapy, it's best for women to consider all their options and make a decision that they individually are most comfortable with, according to their own bodies.

The Power of Testosterone

Often referred to as the hormone of desire, testosterone has the power to make us feel sexual and lusty. Sexually, the presence of testosterone is not only linked to sexual desire but also to feelings of well-being and a sense of energy in men and women. When we don't have enough testosterone, we often feel sluggish about sex or lose interest in it completely.

TESTOSTERONE AND MEN

When testosterone levels are high or adequate, men feel alive, vigorous, and sexually tuned in and frequently turned on. However, testosterone, which is produced by the testicles, decreases gradually and variably with age. At low levels not only can the male experience diminished libido, but also difficulty attaining an erection. Of course this is not the sole cause or even the most frequent reason for loss of erections, but measuring levels of testosterone in the blood or saliva is an important step in understanding any kind of erectile problem. Since testosterone cannot be readily absorbed from the stomach in pill form, skin patches and creams are applied to hairless areas of a man's body, such as the back, abdomen, and buttocks.

However, it is important to keep in mind that replacement of testosterone requires a careful analysis of the libido and/or the erectile problem. Because testosterone can stimulate prostatic growth, an evaluation of the size of the prostate as well as measurement of the PSA (prostatic specific antigen) is required before this hormone is given to a man. Another concern is the correlation of testosterone with levels of cholesterol in the blood. If your total cholesterol and LDL cholesterol, the "bad" lipid, are high, you need to remain observant and check in with your physician regularly. This is also true of watching liver function—your physician may recommend a liver function test during treatment.

By now, most of us know that women also have and need testosterone. The ovaries produce about one third to one half of this hormone, while adrenal gland production accounts for the rest. There is definite variation in the amount of testosterone from woman to woman, and there is a decrease in production as women enter the menopausal transition. When women lose this hormone they experience not only loss of sexual desire, but also decreased sexual responsiveness. They complain of clitoral numbness, atrophy, and difficulty being orgasmic.

Interestingly, women can begin to lose testosterone before the actual onset of menopause. This may result in a woman suddenly losing her desire for sex or having trouble reaching orgasm when she had no problem before, and she may be at a loss to explain the situation. Of course something else in her body or life may be causing these changes, but if it's a loss of testosterone it can be traced. Thankfully, there is a simple blood or saliva test to detect testosterone deficiency.

An often overlooked group of women who experience low desire that can be directly linked to hormones are those who have had an oophorectomy (removal of the ovaries). When the ovaries are removed, usually along with the entire uterus, most gynecologists are very alert to the symptoms of estrogen lack. Often, an estrogen patch is placed on the patient in the recovery room to ease the transition from having functioning ovaries to nothing. Equally as often testosterone deficiency is ignored. Some women, however, do continue to make plenty of this hormone despite the loss of ovarian production. Some individuals have sufficient levels because of adrenal sources. And some women with low levels feel fine. Not every menopausal woman needs this hormone. Also, there can be side effects to deal with, such as acne, edgy mood, facial hair growth, or blood cholesterol changes. Usually, these side effects are not seen at low levels of replacement, but they must be watched for as treatment is initiated. Replacement doses can and should be individualized in an effort to fine-tune the regimen for optimal sense of well-being, lean muscle mass, and libido.

The good news is that the more doctors and researchers focus on women's sexuality and its relation to hormones, the more we will know about the subtleties of testosterone replacement. A testosterone patch for women is currently being tested. Then, when accurate studies and tests have been done, we can all look forward to a future where women will no longer face blank stares as they discuss libido and vitality with their doctors.

Progesterone—An Important Balance

Progesterone is produced in a woman's ovary by the egg sac that is left behind after a ripened egg has erupted at ovulation each month and prepares the uterine lining for the fertilized egg that nature hopes for. In fact, if there is insufficient progesterone for this function, even the most perfectly dividing, fertilized egg will have no place to implant after its trip down the fallopian tube from the ovary. Lack of progesterone is therefore one of the causes of infertility.

On the other hand, if there is no fertilization, the progesterone production is quickly exhausted. When the level of progesterone falls, the lining of the uterus begins to separate and is shed as a woman's monthly period. This is all well and good. However, progesterone/estrogen imbalance can wreak havoc with other body systems producing the notorious PMS, or premenstrual syndrome, as well as breast tenderness, bloating, and irritability.

But what is important for women is to retain a healthy estrogen/progesterone balance. The perimenopausal woman who is still having periods but making less estrogen than she used to may be able to use a low-dose estrogen patch the week before she bleeds in order to balance the progesterone when it is at its highest. The woman who is menopausal and on a prescribed cycle can increase her dose of estrogen by half during the days she is taking the progesterone.

Again, taking any hormonal replacement is a very personal decision that you must review with a trusted physician. Please pay attention to new studies and research, as this field is wide open and constantly changing.

Medications That Impact Sexual Functioning

The list of drugs that adversely affect sexual functioning is huge. Almost any and all medications have been reported at one time or another to cause sexual difficulty. So, if you were doing fine until you started a new drug, be sure to ask your physician if there is a history of similar problems linked to this drug, and/or see if there is another drug that you could try for the problem.

I have gathered here a fairly complete list of the most common medications, their general categories, and how they may affect women.

Medications That May Contribute to Sexual Disorders in Women

(Listed by drug name with trade name in parentheses)

Impact: D/D = decreased desire

ANTIHYPERTENSIVES (TREAT HIGH BLOOD PRESSURE)

Clonidine (Catapres)—inhibition of orgasm

Methyldopa (Aldomet)—D/D, inhibition of orgasm

Propranolol (Inderal)—D/D

Reserpine—D/D

Spironolactone (Aldactone)—D/D; it's also a diuretic, so it causes decreased lubrication

Timolol (Blocadren) (also treats glaucoma)—D/D

ANTIDEPRESSANTS (TREAT DEPRESSION)

Bupropion (Wellbutrin)—D/D

Fluoxetine (Prozac)—D/D, lack of orgasm

Imipramine (Tofranil, Janimine)—D/D, or delayed orgasm

Paroxetine (Paxil)—no orgasm

Sertraline (Zoloft)—delayed or no orgasm

Trazodone (Desyrel)—in rare cases, increased desire

ANTIANXIETY MEDICATIONS (TREAT ANXIETY)

Alprazolam (Xanax)—D/D; inhibition of orgasm

Barbituates—D/D

Diazepam (Valium, Zetran)—delayed or no orgasm

Fluphenazine (Prolixin, Permitil)—D/D

Lithium (Eskalith, Lithonate), also treats bipolar disorder—D/D

Prochlorperazine (Compazine)—decreased responsiveness

ANTIPSYCHOTIC MEDICATIONS (TREAT PSYCHOSIS)

Clomipramine (Anafranil)—D/D, inhibition of orgasm

ILLICIT AND ABUSED DRUGS

Alcohol—D/D or delayed orgasm

Amphetamines—inhibition of orgasm

Diazepam (Valium)—delayed or no orgasm

MDMA—inhibited orgasm

Methaqualone—D/D

NONPRESCRIPTION MEDICATIONS

Cimetidine (Tagemet HB)—D/D

Diphenhydramine (Benadryl)—D/D

Niacin (B3)—D/D

Ranitidine (Zantac 75)—D/D

MISCELLANEOUS MEDICATIONS

Ethinyl estradiol (Estinyl) (birth control pill)—D/D

Fenfluramine (Fastin)—D/D frequent in women with large
    doses or long-term use.

Ketoconazole (Nizoral) (treats yeast infections)—D/D

Levodopa (Larodopa, Dopar)—increased desire

Methadone (Dolophine) (treats morphine drug addiction)—
    D/D, no orgasm

Phendimetrazine (Adphen, Bacarate, Anorex, Statobex)—D/D

Phentermine (Fastin, Ionamin)—delayed or no orgasm

Phenytoin (Dilantin) (treats seizures)—D/D

Primidone (Mysoline) (treats seizures)—D/D

STDs (Sexually Transmitted Diseases)

Sexually transmitted diseases may not directly impact orgasms, per se, but they certainly wreak havoc on our sexuality in general. As I mention in my two other books, sexually transmitted diseases can be contracted by anyone having unprotected sex. In fact, one in every fifteen Americans will contract a sexually transmitted disease this year and one in every four Americans already has one. You are not immune by virtue of your age, ethnicity, education, profession, or socioeconomic status. What further complicates matters is the fact that it is often difficult to tell who has an STD; many people who are infected look and feel fine and can be blissfully unaware they are infected. For women especially, many STDs have no obvious symptoms until there is already irreparable damage (this is true of chlamydia and pelvic inflammatory disease). Quite often, women are not given the tragic news until they want to start a family and learn that an asymptomatic STD has robbed them of that right, unless they use reproductive technologies, such as in vitro.

STDs can be spread through vaginal, oral, and anal sex. Some can also be spread through any contact between the penis, vagina, mouth, or anus—even without intercourse. If your physician confirms your suspicions, follow the medication instructions to the letter, and tell your partner or partners immediately. There is no question that this can be difficult. But, if your partner is not treated, too, he or she can easily give it back to you or give it to someone else, as well as be at risk of having irreparable damage.

It is not wise, under any circumstances, to self-diagnose

when it comes to personal health. Several of these symptoms can be caused by things other than an STD, and many STDs can exist for a very long time before *any* symptoms are noticeable. If you think you have an STD, see your doctor.

I have listed in the appendix the most common sexually transmitted diseases along with their symptoms, potential dangers, and treatments and/or cures. This list is for your general information. For more information about these and other sexually transmitted diseases, you can call the National STD Hotline at (800) 227-8922. These diseases impact all of your sexuality, not just your orgasm. But as I like to say, better safe than sorry.

Maintaining your sexual health should be equal in importance to maintaining your overall physical and emotional health. Stress is unavoidable, but there are ways to keep the channels of awareness open. If you are not functioning at your sexual peak, you can at the very least feel confident and assured that you are able to achieve this necessary health. Sex is too important to give up or compromise.

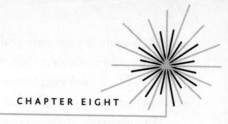

CHAPTER EIGHT

The Beauty of Enhancers

The Wide Angle on Sex and Orgasms

B y this stage of the book, you could probably guess that in my opinion great, mind-blowing sex does not occur in only one position or manner, much less is it tied strictly to intercourse in the missionary position. I'm not only an advocate of bringing oral and manual techniques into the bedroom but also of enhancing your sexual pleasure in any way possible, or at least, in any way with which you are comfortable. Of course there are toys, and in doing my sexuality seminars the past few years since the publication of my first book I have noticed that more and more couples seem to be curious about or have already begun experimenting with some fabulous little (and not so little) gizmos. More on that later. But enhancing your sexual response is not limited to toys. There are many and varied ways to awaken your bodies and build more intense and broad sensation. And while all this stimulation may lead to an orgasm, orgasm is not the only goal here. Then again, if a quickie orgasm is your only goal, you might want to disregard all of this information for the time being.

However, if fabulous, mind-blowing sex is your goal, then you might want to pay attention. I'm also going to give you tips on aromatherapy stimulants and more practical information on supposed aphrodisiacs. The skinny? Some work, some don't. I have also gathered some tips on lubricants so you can add lots of wet and wild pleasures to improve your orgasmic control and degree of pleasure.

> **HISTORICAL AND HYSTERICAL FACTS**
>
> The Marquesans were one of the few peoples whose women controlled the sexual relationship. At feasts, which generally turned into orgies, the males sucked the females' breasts and performed cunnilingus. When the women felt prepared, they demanded intercourse.

The Swirl and Sensual Massage

Most of us can still remember the thrill of heavy petting. The groping, the teasing, the waiting, the working around the hot spots of our bodies when we were teenagers and not really supposed to be "going all the way." A lot of that thrill came from having to stay away from directly touching the genitals. I like to use this technique of anticipation in as many ways as possible: the hotter you are before genital stimulation, the more intense the orgasm will be. Don't forget: This is an age when many women first experienced breast and mouth orgasms as a result of that intense stimulation. One man told me that having his nipples played with felt like "kryptonite. I get completely weak and she knows just how to tweak them. It's like an electric shock to my penis. That in combination with an all-over chest massage, I am done. She doesn't even have to touch Johnny anymore."

As I've been describing throughout this book, the body is full of erogenous zones. Awakening the body is the first step to eliciting sexual pleasure and opening the possible avenues to orgasm. I suggest two specific techniques that couples can use on each other to warm and excite.

THE SWIRL

With either your nails or your fingertips, move along her body (or his if you are the woman) in wavy, undulating strokes from the feet up toward the groin area. Or you can start at her head or shoulders and move down toward her groin. Either way, the slow, undulating wave of touch is creating tingles of sensation without directly touching her genitals. With a straight-line motion, the nerves know when they will be next. With a wavy, irregular pattern, there's more anticipation and the little nerves hope that they're next.

SECRET FROM LOU'S ARCHIVES

Scientists now know why touching is so therapeutic. Massage has been shown to trigger the release of oxytocin in the brain. The hormone produces feelings of sedation and relaxation, lowers blood pressure, and creates a metabolic environment that encourages the storage of nutrients and stimulates growth.

THE SENSUAL MASSAGE

Here I will give what I like to call the sensual massage primer. This particular move is best used as a form of foreplay, when you are trying to arouse each other before you directly involve your genitals. Using both hands, gently but steadily apply pressure to the different parts of his or her body. I think it's always best to start at the top and work down toward the feet. Don't include the groin area for either of you, and avoid her breasts. These areas are much too sensitive; the idea here is to keep each other at a comfortable hum of sexual tension—not go over the top. Now continue pressuring the body as you move down or up, kneading the muscles lightly or deeply, depending on how much pressure he or she prefers. You might also keep in mind that your strokes can either go with the muscles or against them, if a stronger sensation is preferred. Here are some other tips:

> ➤ Probably the most important thing to remember is to maintain continuity and go slowly. The body seems to love surprise sensations that create pleasure, but only if the moves are comfortable and in the range of familiar. Do not go from head to thighs, arms to feet. Rather, move down one side of the body gradually, using big strokes at first and then moving to smaller strokes.
> ➤ Always balance what you do on one side by repeating the move on the other side.
> ➤ Use motions that move the blood toward the heart or away from the heart.
> ➤ Start with broader sensations and strokes and finish each area with soft, light touches.

➤ Use lotion or massage oil so that your hands move easily over the skin. Reapply as necessary.

➤ Make sure your hands are warm; if not, rub them together briskly.

➤ Use a towel or sheet to cover parts of the body you are not touching, so she or he stays warm.

Aromatherapy

Aromatherapy can be used to not only enhance moods but to induce moods, from relaxed, romantic, and sensual to heightened sexual states. For those of you interested in creating your own aromatherapy wardrobe, you might consider the recipes for essential-oil combination that are said to induce some of the responses listed below, or see the chart on pages 186–187 for a thorough listing.

Mildly sedative—chamomile, sandalwood, lavender, vetiver

Alertness—black pepper, rosemary, lemon, peppermint

Normalizing effect—bergamot and lavender

Predispose mind and body to sexual ecstasy—vaporized oil of frankincense

During the course of writing this book, I had the unique opportunity to become my own guinea pig to test the impact of aromatherapy. I can certainly attest to the efficacy of the lemongrass-rosemary combination, which helped my mental clarity. I used a small water-style diffuser with a votive candle, which smelled delightful. When I started getting fuzzy, I'd refresh the scent, make a cup of herbal tea, and walk around my

Essential Aromatherapy Oils

FOR WOMEN	FOR MEN

FOR IMPROVING YOUR MOOD

FOR WOMEN	FOR MEN
Jasmine: enhances femininity	Vanilla: unleashes deep emotion and hidden sexuality
Chamomile (B): clears emotional debris	
Neroli: intensely female	Orange (A): helps sort out emotional tangles
Grapefruit: for a liquid face-lift; brightens things	

SEXUALLY REGULATING AND STIMULATING

FOR WOMEN	FOR MEN
Bergamot (B): enlivens sex life	Cardamon: evokes the exotic nature
Geranium (B): balances; creates harmony between the sexes	Vetivert: sexually arousing and stimulating

APHRODISIACS

FOR WOMEN	FOR MEN
Ylang-ylang: intense exotic (however, in large doses it has the opposite effect)	Sandalwood: profoundly masculine; a sedative; seductive
Jasmine: empress; 100 percent feminine	Clary Sage (C): a sexual opiate
Clary Sage (C): like a seductive man	Patchouli: associated with ancient eroticism, earthy
Rose: enlivens your heart	Cumin: a powerful stimulant for the flow of body juices

FOR AN INVIGORATING ENERGY BOOST

FOR WOMEN	FOR MEN
Lemongrass: clean, lively	Juniper: a sexy oil
Rosemary (B): increases creativity, lifts exhaustion	Ginger (A, B): inviting and arousing

Essential Aromatherapy Oils

FOR WOMEN	FOR MEN

FOR INCREASING MENTAL ACUITY; STRENGTHENS MEMORY

FOR WOMEN	FOR MEN
Melissa: gentle, soft; good when suffering from mental exhaustion	Black Pepper: promotes stamina and strength (use sparingly)
Rosemary (B): royal in stature; stimulates sensitivity	Bay: stimulates imagination; not for the submissive!

RELAXING, REGULATING, SOOTHING

FOR WOMEN	FOR MEN
Lavender: steadying influence	Frankincense: releases subconscious stress
Marjoram: for when you need a cuddle, not sex	Cinnamon: sensually calming for nerves

HOW TO USE

For all: through vaporizing, mixed with oil for massage, or in a bath. Or: as a mouthwash (A); as a hot (B) or cold (C) compress.

FOR A FACIAL MASSAGE

Dilute 15 drops of chosen essential oil in 1 ounce almond oil. Use an oil appropriate for your skin type.

SKIN TYPE	OIL
Dry	Sandalwood, Rose
Sensitive	Chamomile, Lavender
Oily	Lavender, Ylang-Ylang
Normal	Geranium, Neroli

home for a few minutes while the scent spread throughout the rooms.

Scented candles or incense also work to create relaxation. You may want to try patchouli, ylang-ylang, and vanilla, which are popular scents, as well as clary sage, rose, and geranium.

The reason aromatherapy is so effective is that the scent detected by the olfactory nerve impacts the brain immediately, unlike other substances you may drink or eat, which have to pass through the blood before they fully impact the body.

SECRET FROM LOU'S ARCHIVES

A woman's sense of smell is more keen than a man's due to her higher levels of estrogen. As Marc McCutcheon points out, women can detect the odor of musk—a scent associated with male bodies—better than any other odor. When estrogen levels peak during ovulation, a woman's sense of smell is more acute and can detect musk one hundred times more keenly.

Aphrodisiacs

There are a number of myths about aphrodisiacs, and some of these age-old products work, while others are pure hooey. For the record (as I mention above), such products as essential oils (in the form of candles, incense, or bath foams) can and do increase libido, simply because they relax you and put you in the mood.

A definition of "aphrodisiac" according to Brenda Love, author of *Encyclopedia of Unusual Sex Practices*, is "a chemical that increases or enhances sexual desire and stamina. The term comes from Aphrodite, the Greek Goddess of Love and Beauty." She then categorizes them into two groups—dietary and drug. Experts believe that the most successful aphrodisiac harmonies are those which are subliminally reminiscent of bodily secretions or excretions. Just about anything can be considered an aphrodisiac if it works on one of your five senses and creates a sexual response. Any image or substance that elicits a response from your sense of taste, smell, hearing, sight, or touch, or any combination made from all of five can be considered an aphrodisiac. Cynthia Mervis Watson, M.D., author of *Love Potions*, states that "when all are stimulated at once, look out!"

Aphrodisiacs have taken the shape of food or drink, herb or spice, charm or ritual, drug, homeopathic remedy, flower essence or aroma. Although they varied in form, aphrodisiacs were among ancient cultures' great common denominators: remedies promising similar results have been found in China, Egypt, Mesopotamia, India, Europe, Africa, South America, and Polynesia.

The bottom line is, if you think they work, they will. Certain substances like oysters, which contain zinc, are a potent mineral for sexual functioning in men. Also, it is interesting to note that oysters resemble female genitalia.

According to Watson, certain aphrodisiacs are "really simple as high school chemistry." The body is able to manufacture hormones, neurotransmitters, and neuropeptides only when fed certain essential ingredients. Many traditional aphrodisiacs are high in amino acids and the required enzymes and vitamins, which is why they work. Watson mentions that such plant extracts as yohimbe, spikenard, suma, muira puama, guarana, damiana, saw palmetto, vanilla, wild yam, ginko, bee pollen, and kava kava have been understood to show some aphrodisiac effects.

Some aphrodisiacs, such as the recreational drug MDMA (known by its street name, Ecstasy), work by altering the levels of neurotransmitters and neuropeptides. Ecstasy causes a huge release of serotonin that produces a feeling of euphoria, but at the same time, the drug also inhibits orgasm. Another way aphrodisiacs can work is to act as an MAO (monoamine oxidase) inhibitor. That means it inhibits the production of the substance that recycles neurotransmitters, so their concentration increases in the body.

Lubricants

Where would we be without lubricant? Ladies, you can't always expect yourselves to be wet and wild; and, gentlemen, I know you'll love the soft, slinky pleasure that lube adds to your lady, her toys, and her fingers! Using lube only increases your pleasure potential. Before we get started, there are a few details you should keep in mind when choosing a personal lubricant:

➤ I recommend using water-based lubricants with condoms; they are safer, come back to life with a quick drop of water, and they will not corrode the latex found in condoms. Although oil-based lubricants are fine for manual sex, if you're planning to continue on to intercourse using a condom, you're kind of stuck. It's best to simply use a lubricant that is water based.

➤ *Always* read the label of a lubricant in its entirety. If you see the word "oil" listed anywhere under ingredients, chances are the product is not water based.

➤ Watch out for the ingredient known as nonoxynol-9. It was originally brought into this country from Germany in the 1930s as a hospital cleaning solution and can be extremely irritating to both men and women. You may also see nonoxynol-9 described as a protectant against HIV yet there are no conclusive studies proving this to date. Dr. Helene Gayle of the CDC (Centers for Disease Control) said that "nonoxynol-9 should not be recommended as an effective means of HIV prevention."

➤ Be careful of anything described as a "body-glide." Eros, Venus, Millenium, and Platinum are four such examples of these body-glides, which are marketed as lubricants. Instead they are made of silicone and carry no protective value and they aren't water soluble. They will have dimenthicone or dimenthiconicol listed on the label.

➤ If the label says it is for external cosmetic use only or for topical cosmetic use only, do not put it anywhere near your delicate tissue—either externally or internally.

➤ Rule of thumb: If a label has "avoid contact with eyes," I might recommend you not use that product genitally, since the sensitive mucosal tissue of your eyes, sinuses, and mouth is almost identical to that of your vulvar genital area. So, as I was told by a gynecologist, "If you wouldn't put it in your eye, do not put it up there either."

➤ Be careful when introducing any colored (dyes) and or scented (flavored) product internally. Consider using externally first and check your sensitivity before using internally, as they can cause yeast and bladder infections. If you are concerned or sensitive, test the production on yourself a day or two in advance of using it.

➤ **Sensura/Sex Grease.** This is the water-based lubricant of choice for many connoisseurs. It is a clear thick liquid with a velvety texture that maintains a slick feel for a long time. The same product is marketed under two different names and in two different packages. For the ladies it is called Sensura and bottled in pink. For the men it is called Sex Grease and bottled in black. It's great for intercourse because of its thick, velvety texture.

➤ **Very Private Intimate Moisturizer.** One of the best new products I have found. The creator behind this product came up with it because she couldn't find a product on the market that met her own needs. She had spent years in the cosmetic business and has now created her own private line, working with dermatologists and gynecologists. This is an outstanding lubricant, especially for women. It actually feels more like a moisturizer in that it doesn't just sit on the surface of your skin but is lightly absorbed. It's water based, colorless and fragrance free. She also created a body wash and a body lotion and they are lovely products. If it's not available in your area, you can order from my website, www.loupaget.com.

➤ **Liquid Silk.** The name describes it all. This creamy water-based British lubricant in a pump bottle contains no glycerine, so it doesn't get sticky. It has become a favorite of field researchers. It is great for manual techniques and intercourse. It does, however, have a slightly bitter taste, which detracts from its use during oral sex.

➤ **Midnite Fire.** This is the product that "snaps open." Midnite Fire is almost guaranteed to bring you lots of enjoyment. It not only comes in a variety of flavors, it also becomes very warm with gentle rubbing and even warmer when you blow on it following the rub. Not to worry, though, the heat only builds to a certain level so there is no risk of getting burned. As with any product, text for your own sensitivity. Midnite Fire is a water-based lubricant that is safe for application both internally and externally. Although it is billed as "The Hot Sensual Massage Lotion," it's really too thick to be used for a straight massage without adding water or another clear water-based lubricant. It feels especially erotic when applied to the nipples, inner thighs, the head of the penis, and the testicles.

SECRET FROM LOU'S ARCHIVES

At the risk of being annoying, I must again warn you to avoid, at all cost, using any lubricant containing nonoxynol-9 during oral sex. This ingredient not only tastes awful, it will have a slight numbing effect on your mouth.

Toys, Toys, Toys

There's no doubt in my mind that toys can add excitement, variety, and intensity to your sex life. I offer you here a quick overview of the favorite toys that men and women in my seminars have used and enjoyed. I also provide information about how to select a dildo or vibrator and how to use them. My first two books offer a more complete listing and description of toys—enough to fill an entire pleasure chest! In the appendix I have listed the places (with either addresses, toll-free phone numbers, or e-mail addresses) where you can order toys.

Though I encourage you to use toys in any way you see fit, I do suggest some Cardinal Toy Rules:

1. You need to keep your toys clean. Wash them in warm water and an antibacterial soap before and after you use your toys.
2. Use only water-based lubricants with any of your plastic-compound items, as oil products, massage oil, or hand lotion (anything containing lanolin or petrolatum) will start to break down the surface of the plastic.
3. Use a condom on parts that are inserted vaginally or anally; this will clean up a lot easier.
4. Keep toys used for different areas (vaginal versus anal) separate from one another. For example, if your partner likes anal penetration, then don't use that dildo for her vagina, and so on. Toy-savvy types have one bag for vaginal toys and another for anal.

5. Keep your toys in a safe place, away from dust and oils.
6. Don't share your toys. Why risk it?

Dildo Basics

There is a style and type of dildo or vibrator to suit everyone—man or woman. Some are completely lifelike, having been molded from real people, often adult film stars.

It's important to choose a style that suits you and one that is easy to clean. Some women prefer those made of silicone because they warm up faster than the latex. Some women enjoy the heightened sensations and contractions of the vagina during climax that come from the PC muscle tightening around the dildo, creating more tension.

You have your choice of:

SIZE:

➤ Sizes range from very small to full arm size. The larger are admittedly for a specialized "niche" market.
➤ With or without "balls."
➤ Double dildos for simultaneous penetration for the two partners.

MATERIAL:

➤ Cyberskin, plastic (hard or soft), latex, silicone, metal, rubber, vinyl, Jelee™.

SHAPE:

➤ Straight, curved, lifelike, ridged, smooth, egg, telescoping, and a special design suitable for G-spot/prostate stimulation.

VIBRATING FEATURES:

➤ Vibrating dildos; typically the vibrating part (which can be adjusted to different pulsations) will be aligned to stimulate the clitoris while the shaft portion is inserted vaginally. Meanwhile, the shaft portion can be doing something nifty such as rotating, twisting at the head, pulsing in and out at the same time the clitoris is being stimulated. Vibration can also be variable pulsations.

➤ Power source from battery or electricity.

COLOR:

➤ Any color you can imagine: fluorescent, black, brown, pink, flesh, clear, purple, white, solids, stripes, sparkles—the list is quite endless.

HARNESSES:

➤ Dildos can be used "freestyle" in your hand or attached to a harness, which is leather or fabric, and worn around your hips.

➤ Thigh harnesses can be used by a man if he wants full-body contact. One seminar attendee told of how her husband, who is paraplegic, fulfilled her beyond her wildest dreams. "He was able to penetrate me in a way I didn't think possible." You never know when these toys will work their magic.

How to Use Them

➤ **Breathe**. As with any sex, breathing is your friend and deep breathing will heighten the sensations.

➤ **Apply to clitoris**. Using a vibrator, have your partner stimulate your clitoris—this will add a significant buzz to partner sex. You can cushion the vibration through a garment or the fleshy outer labia. Often women find direct clitoral stimulation too intense until they are more excited. Use a range of stroking motions up and down the clitoral ridge.

➤ **Insert vaginally**. Insert either a dildo or vibrator in the interior of the vagina; the first 1^1/$_2$ inches is the most sensitive.

➤ **Anally**. For those ladies and their men who enjoy anal play, a small butt plug dildo or a vibrating dildo will send you heavenward. Men who enjoy this typically choose a slim little wand style that can be inserted while he's masturbating or you are manually touching him.

➤ **In combo**. On yourself or with a partner. This can be accomplished by wearing a harnessed dildo. Depending on design, the wearer may have a vaginal plug dildo in the harness for them while the "front loaded" dildo is available to penetrate their partner. This way everyone can have the feeling of fullness.

Types of Vibrators and Dildos

These first few toys are classics, and therefore bear repeating from my previous books. If you happen to be a *Sex and the City* fan, you'll know what I mean.

THE RABBIT PEARL

The design of the Rabbit Pearl lends itself to being able to stimulate both partners at the same time. To ensure maximum stimulation for both, it's best to concentrate the vibration in

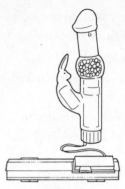

The Rabbit Pearl

the bunny section (leave the articulating option off). This way, the lady can have the wand section inserted vaginally and, with you lying on top of her, your hips matched with hers, turn on the (very strong Japanese) motor. The RP's nose or ears can be stimulating her clitoral area and the back of the Rabbit Pearl can be stimulating the underside of your scrotum.

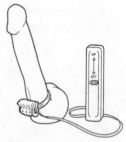

The Microtickler

THE MICRO TICKLER

The small, vibrating silver bullet is encased in an incredibly stretchy sheath that holds it in place at the base of the man. The sheath has a two-textured vibrating surface that can also be used to please a woman.

THE PEARL NECKLACE

I recommend a thirty- to thirty-six-inch strand of 8–10mm round costume pearls because of their smooth, even size and shape. (It's best to use costume pearls, not real, natural pearls.) Lightly lubricate his penis, then slowly adorn him by wrapping the pearls around the shaft. Be sure to hold the necklace clasp with one finger, as you don't want it to scratch and distract him. If you've worn them out for dinner, the pearls will be softly warm. When his penis looks like it is

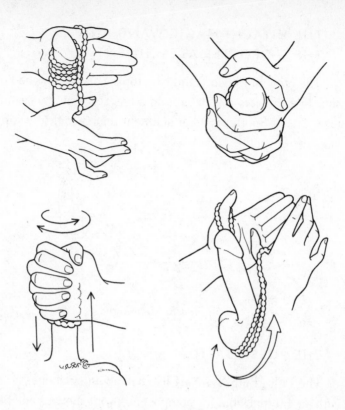

The Pearl Necklace

wearing a Princess Diana choker, start slowly stroking him up and down with the Basket Weave stroke. You can then unwrap his penis and, almost like you are flossing under his testicles, slowly pull the pearls from one side to the other, slightly lifting his testicles. And when you are done you can "coil the poiles" at the base of his shaft and settle yourself on top of him. No doubt pearls will start to have a new place in your repertoire!

THE HITACHI MAGIC WAND AND
THE G-SPOTTER ATTACHMENT

The Hitachi Magic Wand vibrator is a classic for good reason. It stimulates a wide area in a big, soft way that women love. The G-Spotter is an attachment that specifically stimulates the G-spot.

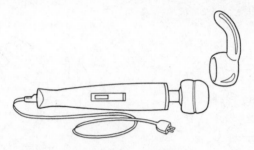

The Hitachi Magic Wand

THE PULSA BATH

The Pulsa Bath is a Nerf-like ball about six inches across with an internal vibrating component—your showers and bath time will never be the same.

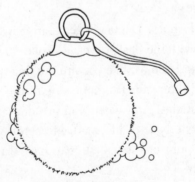

The Pulsa Bath

FINGER VIBE

The Finger Vibe is one of the more powerful, almost silent fingertip vibrator. It is soft, and you can pinpoint the vibration very specifically. It doesn't ever numb your finger—a terrific new product!

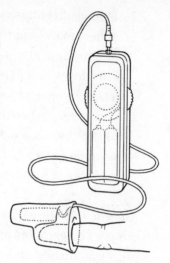

Finger Vibe

COCK RINGS

The theory behind cock rings is the law of hydraulics. An erect penis is a study in hydraulics. Stimulation causes blood to flow in and fill the penis chambers. Gravity and a drop-off of stimulation cause the blood to flow back out. Cock rings work temporarily by greatly reducing the drop-off of penile blood pressure by holding shut the veins along the sides of the erect penis that allow the blood to flow out. The result is a firmer, more long-lasting erection. And some men report delays in ejaculation.

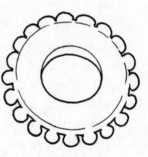

Cock Ring

Here are the ways cock rings can be worn:

1. They can be worn during manual stimulation by either partner and or during intercourse.

2. During intercourse some couples have reported they either enjoyed starting and then removing the ring prior to climax or placing it on halfway through and finishing with it in place.

3. The scrotum and penis may appear to be a much darker color when the ring is in place. That is natural as the blood is pooled there. The ring should not be worn for longer than twenty to thirty minutes without removing it for a few minutes for a break.

Directions: To be most effective, the gentleman, or his partner, applies a light lubricant on the ring and himself. It's best to use a water-based one, as it will not break down the material the way oils or lotions will. It is easiest when he is fully erect, but that state is not necessary. Afterward, merely wash with antibacterial soap and water and it will be ready for next time.

This is a very stretchy material, up to 7". Play with it and see. The correct and most effective position for the ring is to encircle the shaft and underneath the scrotum. Placing it only on the shaft has some men reporting, "It was too tight just on the shaft and yet even though I thought the other way would be more of the same, oddly I felt more supported and 'just right.'"

It's best that the gentleman does the final adjusting over the testicles. Often couples will try the ring first during manual and when they know what works for them they move to intercourse.

One of the most important things about cock rings is the need to put them on correctly—gently over the shaft and scrotum. When used incorrectly, thrusting can be painful. A typical style is made of cloth, metal, plastic, or leather with an adjustable strap to adjust tightness.

SWAROVSKI TEMPORARY CRYSTAL TATTOOS

Stylish, unique, and eye-catching—could you ask for more in an accessory? Easy to apply, available in multiple colors and a broad range of designs, they have become a big hit when applied to publicly viewed areas and to more private spots. Be judicious when you place them—if placed in the pubic triangle area, they can be slightly scratchy during activity. They are crystals after all. They can be worn for two to three days.

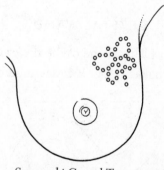

Swarovski Crystal Tattoo

EXERCISING EGGS

These solid marble eggs can be inserted vaginally and used by women so they can concentrate on the sensation of resist-

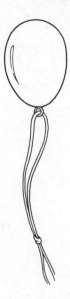

ance to the egg. The idea behind any instrument or exercise that strengthens the PC muscle is to give a woman a more refined physical awareness of what her muscles are doing and how they are feeling. Some women like to warm up the egg first by running it under warm water. Also, you need to cleanse it before and after use with hot soapy water. One can practice letting the egg drop and then concentrate on contracting and pulling it up the vaginal vault. There is a string attached for easy removal (similar to a tampon). For those who are interested, Mantak Chia, in his book *Cultivating Female Sexual Energy* offers a whole

Exercising Egg chapter of different exercises.

CRYSTAL WAND

This is one of the better G-spot stimulating devices and it makes sense. It is designed by a woman. Made of solid, clear

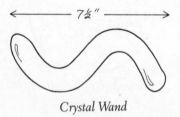

Crystal Wand

acrylic, it can be angled and rested on a pillow so that the woman can maintain the pressure she prefers while masturbating. It can also be used by a man for prostate stimulation.

The ever-ingenious Chinese created sexual toys in the twelfth and thirteenth centuries such as the double olishos, a dildo that could accommodate two women at once. The device was contained in an ivory or wooden phallus with two silk belts in the middle of it. The movement of one woman created pleasure for the other. Another device was a dildo that could be manipulated by moving the heel of the foot. This kept the hands free for other amorous activities, or perhaps household duties.

Surgical Procedures

There are certain surgical procedures that promise to increase control or intensity of orgasms in men and women. And while some of these are gaining popular attention, I can only recommend a few, as the others are quite dangerous or create very serious side effects.

The surgical enhancement procedures for men concern penis enlargement and there are two main types of surgeries: (1) the cutting of the suspensory ligaments that attach the root of the penis to the pelvis, which causes the penis to drop and hence have a longer look when flaccid. Unfortunately, this makes the erection less stable because its support structures have been cut; (2) the injection of the man's adipose (fat) tissue that has been harvested from another area of his body. The adipose tissue is injected into the penis to increase its width. The problem with this procedure is the tendency to reabsorb the adipose in an irregular fashion, leaving the man with a lumpy penis. One woman referred to a penis that underwent this procedure as "a swollen angry sausage."

I agree with Drs. Milsten and Slowinski, who approach these types of procedures with an "if it ain't broke, don't fix it" attitude. As described above, these procedures are often fraught with problems and may not be worth the pain of surgery.

Also important to know is how other kinds of surgery can impact your sexual functioning. For instance, if a hysterectomy is necessary, then a woman should ask her doctor to make sure that the cuff of skin at the neck of the cervix where it protrudes into the vagina is left so her orgasmic response stays intact. When the entire uterus is removed, there is a lessening of orgasmic response, which makes sense, as the nerves associated with being able to register and deliver sensation are gone. The lesson here is this: Stop the number of unnecessary hysterectomies. They may be good for surgeons' bank accounts, but they are bad for women and their partners as well.

Men will also want to know that prostate surgery (as treatment in the event of prostate cancer) now typically includes nerve-sparing techniques. This is so the bundle of nerves (the prostatic plexus) that passes over the lateral side of the prostate are not cut and removed along with the prostate as a matter of course. When the nerves are left intact as much as possible, a man can maintain more of his potency. It may take a bit for the sensation of the surgically disturbed nerves to return, but they invariably do.

Exercises

There are different exercises that will increase your degree of pleasure. The most common and talked-about exercise is of course the Kegel, which directly strengthens and tones the PC (pubococcygeal) muscles in both women and men. The PC muscle is your sex muscle. For women, it is essentially the floor of their entire pelvic region, holding up the uterus, the anus, the entire urinary tract. It also is directly connected to the clitoris, which as we saw earlier has very long legs, capable of carrying waves of pleasure as if it were a telephone wire. Strengthening and toning the PC muscle not only prevents incontinence later in life but also allows you to feel deeper, longer-lasting orgasms. As Dr. Beverly Whipple attests, there is a direct correlation between a well-toned PC muscle and the intensity of orgasms in men and women.

Kegels

Doing Kegels also can make the entire vaginal entry firmer, which heightens sensation for women and is a quality most men absolutely enjoy. The two muscle groups that make up the female pelvic floor are the outermost near the clitoris and the urethral sphincter muscles. The second group is made up of the inner rear muscles near the anus and includes the pubococcygeus, iliococcygeus, and the levator ani muscles.

The exercise:

➤ Lie supine, knees flexed, feet flat.
➤ Place one hand on the floor, and rest the other on your abdomen.

- Contract and internally lift the region between your genitals and anus, squeezing your muscles inward, toward the center of your body.
- Breathe in and out as you squeeze and release the muscle.
- If you are a woman, you can test the tightness of this muscle by inserting your finger about two inches into the vagina and squeezing as if you were stopping the flow of urine.

For men, the PC muscle functions in an analogous way, and strengthening it can also increase potency. While erect, contract your PC muscle and watch it jump. To increase the resistance (as a strengthener), you can use a wet washcloth draped over your erect penis in the shower or afterward.

Another larger, more general way to enhance your entire sexual experience, especially your orgasm, is by utilizing sexual techniques from the East, namely Tantra, which approaches sex as a path to enlightenment through exquisite awareness and control of the body. We Westerners can adapt some of these ancient techniques and give our sexual experience a heightened, spiritual dimension.

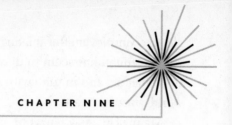

CHAPTER NINE

Sex and the Spirit

Transforming Sexual Energy into Spiritual Love

Sex can be fun. Sex can be passionate. Sex can be physically pleasurable. Sex can also be spiritual. If you think about it, every event in our lives—whether it be a drive in the car, a game of golf, or a making love—can be experienced three ways: physically, emotionally, and spiritually. Sometimes these elements fuse together, making an event that much more meaningful. Yet for many of us, and I include myself in this category, spirituality was the domain of organized religion, and in most cases that didn't include an open, passionate view of sexuality. The main message received about sex coming through these channels tended to be that sex and religion simply don't mix. A bit like dogs circling each other, each camp saw the other as an adversary, possibly acknowledging the existence of the other but staying distant.

This chapter is for those readers who want to feel connected with their partner in a spiritual way—perhaps not all the time, but at least once in a while. Have you ever felt so close to your lover after making love or during an orgasm that your surroundings seem to disappear? You and your lover are so connected and in tune with each other that the rest of the world ceases to matter?

Many of us may have one memory of such an experience when sex transported us to another realm. This sometimes occurs only with one person and fleetingly, but it is experienced as a hugely different connection and state during lovemaking. Some of the masters of spiritual sexuality refer to this state as ecstasy and think of it as the supreme form of making love. But how and why does this happen? For those of us who have had this experience, it seems to have come out of nowhere, a spontaneous event that is completely out of our control. Or is it in our control?

SECRET FROM LOU'S ARCHIVES

According to Margot Anand, the five virtues of the ecstatic lover are: Patience, Trust, Presence, Compassion, and Clarity.

Sexologist Jack Morin, in his book *The Erotic Mind*, succinctly summarizes why peak erotic experiences are perfectly suited to spiritual experience and transcendence: "They engage us totally, enlarge our sense of self by connecting us with another or with normally hidden dimensions of ourselves or both, and expand our perceptions and consciousness" (as quoted in *Liberated Orgasm* by Herbert Otto). Therapists Jack Zimmerman and Jaquelyn McCandless have termed this "expanded state of awareness" the Third Presence. In their own relationship, they experienced a distinctive state of awareness made possible by the transcendent spiritual dimension of their relationship. As they describe in their book, *Flesh and Spirit*, "What we are really talking about [is] an expanded state of consciousness that is co-created by two partners together with something unconditional and ultimately mysterious that is not of the ordinary world."

In this country, there has been interest in a sacred form of sex since the 1960s, and this growing interest in the spiritual then evolved into the New Age movement. The desire to learn about Eastern philosophies and religions was fueled by two forces: a quest for spiritual knowledge coupled with a rejection of past social and religious limitations on sexual expression. The 1960s radicals who were becoming champions of "free love" wanted to redefine sex and disassociate it from guilt and the concept of sin. They saw sex as an event that celebrated life.

In many ways, this emerging American vision of the new sexuality was borrowing from and building upon what the ancient Eastern schools had believed in for centuries. Specifically, the philosophic schools of Chinese Taoism and Buddhist Tantra had been practicing a sexuality that was very tied to the spiritual realm. These ancient Eastern systems of spiritual enlightenment had their beginnings about 5000 B.C. according to scholars. These groups insist that getting to the spiritual realm through sex is not only possible, it's also probable and a goal one should seek to attain. In fact, they have come up with elaborate ceremonies (over sixty-five different positions) that basically teach you how to enter the "holy realm."

The starting premise is the different natures of men and women and that sexual acts have the capacity to be not only physiologically transportive but psychologically and emotionally enlightening as well. The only requirement is that both partners are in agreement and they proceed in a meditative, studied way.

All Tantra Is Not Created Equal

In the past few years an East-meets-West zeitgeist has brought everything from yoga to Zen Buddhism into mainstream American culture. It seems only natural, then, that we Westerners would also be curious about the Eastern approach to sex, which has as its hallmark a more spiritual point of view. Specifically, Tantra, which developed as a form of yoga practice, embodies this Eastern (both Buddhist and Hindu) ideal. The focus of Tantra is not on transformation of sex, but on the use of sexual energy to develop and create a spiritual experience. Tantric sex uses traditional rituals and specific sex positions to help practitioners achieve mystical union. Tantric practitioners believe in combining relaxation with high states of sexual excitement. Sexual energy is recirculated for an extended time. As a result, there are sometimes long-lasting orgasms, which are not genitally focused.

However, as with most things we import from faraway lands and cultures, some things about Tantra have been lost in translation. As a result, there are many misconceptions about Tantra, ranging from people thinking it's a form of "naked yoga" in which "couples have sex," to people believing that it's merely a form of sexual massage.

Tantra, in its very nature, is viewed as a spiritual exercise and path to enlightenment. Its movements and postures are based on yoga principles of body alignment, and breathing exercises to cleanse the body, mind, and soul. Yet its overall goal maintains that sex leads to achieving a higher level of awareness and connection to the universe, or God. Doing Tantra with your partner becomes a spiritual exercise in which together you bond so deeply that you become one, and nearer to the essence of life.

Tantric students fine-tune their senses so that each becomes one with the universe and with their partner. The exchange of secretions between the man and the woman plays an important role in this process. Three distinct types of sexual secretions or elixirs are produced by the woman—from the breasts, mouth, and yoni (vagina). Absorption by the man of these elixirs is said to be spiritually nourishing and compensates him for the loss of semen, which he gives to the woman. In Tantric practices, the man becomes the Shiva (the Divine Will), which manifests in the creative union with the Shakti (representing pure energy). The woman becomes the Shakti and embodies the fundamental secret forces that control the universe.

Orgasm is usually understood only in physical terms: as a highly pleasurable, explosive-like experience with muscular pelvic contractions most often resulting from stimulation of the genitals. As I've pointed out in the preceding chapters, you don't have to be stimulated genitally to have an orgasm. And just as the genitals should not limit the source of your orgasm, neither should your body limit your experience of an orgasm. The main requirement for accessing this spiritual realm is that you are open and willing to let go of any attitudes that may be holding you back. I promise, this is much easier than it may seem to you at first.

When you approach sex as a spiritual activity, you view orgasm as an exchange of energy between lovers. This exchange creates yet another form of energy that can transform you and your experience, making you feel one with your lover. At the physical level, most of these practices maintain that if a man controls his ejaculation, he will be able to prolong and heighten pleasure for both his partner and himself. Sexologists Marilyn Fithian and William Hartman speculate that the quick intercourse couples often experience "does not allow enough time for the natural chemicals that accompany touch and sexual arousal to be released into the bloodstream, which then short-circuits the general sense of well-being that usually accompanies lovemaking" (as quoted in Chia). In other words, when sex is "hasty," the man and the woman are not able to exchange sexual energy and harmonize with each other, and may even drain each other of energy.

Meditation and breathing techniques are used to control and extend the arousal period so that the penis stays functional for nearly an hour. Now, that might be a nice thing to learn, don't you agree? Based upon these general premises, a couple then has many positions with which they can regulate the flow of energy between each other, and I will address these positions below. It's also important to maintain eye contact and match breathing in order to further connect with your partner. As you may imagine, this is a very subtle process and one that requires both people to be in a calm, relaxed state of mind.

For me, there's a lot about Tantra that is wonderful, transforming, and simply practical. What I've done for you, then, is given you (boiled down) what I think is the best of Tantra. I've streamlined this presentation and left out a lot of the overly "woo-woo" language, without, I hope, losing its spiritual essence. My reason for this is twofold: Many of the books out there on Tantra seem weighted down by too many ideas and New Age gobbledy-gook, which keeps women and men from experiencing, understanding, or using the very practical suggestions for how to improve their sex lives, specifically in the orgasm department.

HISTORICAL AND HYSTERICAL FACTS	Extraordinary sexual positions and entanglements can be seen frozen on ancient Indian temple walls. These positions were created and performed by Tantric holy women trained from childhood in the art of love. For Western Tantrikas, without such a background, these complex positions are difficult and less than comfortable.

Second, though classic Tantra is a form of yoga practice, you don't have to become a yogi to benefit from the movements and exercises. It's my feeling that the more practical, accurate information you have about sex, the more you are likely to grow, explore, and discover sexual satisfaction. So consider this information on Tantra and go to town. To those who are open to new ideas, I guarantee you will learn something about yourself, your body, and how to increase your own and your partner's pleasure quotient.

Lou's Practical Guide to Spiritual Sex

Whatever your personal philosophy or religion, you can still take advantage of the underlying concepts and practice of spiritual sex. That is, if you have the right attitude. As I say above, the "right attitude" is one that is open and willing to the *possibility* of spiritual sex. So before I give you the techniques and positions, I would like to share with you the guidelines that experts say will enable you to reach a heightened and expanded state of awareness and sensation. These guidelines are made up of ideas, which in turn make up the open-minded attitude:

1. Have the same intention. As this is more of a mind-body connection, ideally both partners should have the same intention about their sexual joining. If not, a transportive connection cannot be achieved.
2. Accept your vulnerability. This approach to sex tends to make women and men feel more emotionally vulnerable because it stresses a more passive, receptive state. This is especially true of the man's role to encourage and give to the woman.
3. Set aside enough time during which you will not be

interrupted. Maintaining a soothing, open ambience is crucial to the spiritual-sexual connection.

4. Know that like any new venture it will take time to become proficient. For those who are already comfortable and safe emotionally, you may enter this realm overnight. For others, it may take some time, confidence, and reassurance with your partner.

5. Keep in mind the goal of spiritual sex: connecting spiritually with your partner through sex. This is a sexual attitude and style, not a sexual performance goal. If your only reason to study these philosophies is to discover the way to be multiorgasmic, then you are missing the larger point!

For those who feel these states may not be possible for them, I would like to point out it is easier *done* than *said*. In other words, you may find the language of Tantra a bit new and therefore off-putting, but in practice the actual positions and techniques are quite simple and straightforward. You might also be interested in knowing that the benefits of Tantra are quite real and concrete. Margot Anand points out in her book *Sexual Ecstasy* that Tantric sex can help women

➤ learn the ability to become sexually aroused more quickly and fully;

➤ learn how to experience a whole-body orgasm through sexual intercourse;

and help men

➤ learn to increase their ability to control ejaculation in states of high arousal;

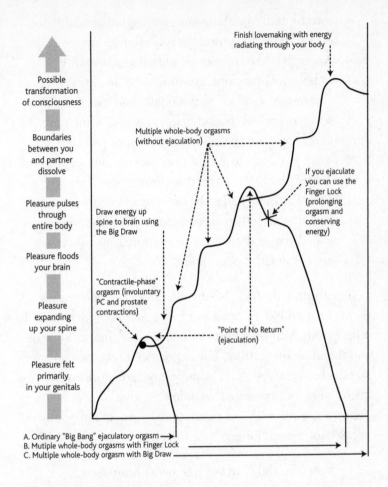

Possible transformation of consciousness

Boundaries between you and partner dissolve

Pleasure pulses through entire body

Pleasure floods your brain

Pleasure expanding up your spine

Pleasure felt primarily in your genitals

Finish lovemaking with energy radiating through your body

Multiple whole-body orgasms (without ejaculation)

Draw energy up spine to brain using the Big Draw

If you ejaculate you can use the Finger Lock (prolonging orgasm and conserving energy)

"Contractile-phase" orgasm (involuntary PC and prostate contractions)

"Point of No Return" (ejaculation)

A. Ordinary "Big Bang" ejaculatory orgasm →
B. Multiple whole-body orgasms with Finger Lock
C. Multiple whole-body orgasm with Big Draw

MALE ORGASMIC POTENTIAL

Instead of the ordinary "Big Bang" ejaculatory orgasm (A), with sexual kung fu you can draw your sexual energy up during contractile phase (before ejaculation) and have multiple whole-body orgasms. If you ejaculate, you can use the Finger Lock, which will prolong your orgasm and conserve energy (B). If you avoid ejaculation, you can use the Big Draw to finish lovemaking with energy radiating through your body (C).

—from *The Multi-Orgasmic Man*, Mantak Chia

➤ learn how to experience extended, whole-body orgasm without ejaculation;

➤ and to experience their full orgasmic potential, as shown in the diagram opposite.

The Basic Positions

Many of the truly ancient Tantric positions are complicated and elaborate and would be difficult to practice by ordinary people on an ordinary day. Charles and Caroline Muir, who have spent years studying and adapting Tantra for Western women and men, have developed five basic sexual positions for people wanting to try Tantra. Within these five positions, hundreds of variations are possible. The five are:

1. Yab Yum, which is unique to Tantra
2. Horizontal with man on top
3. Horizontal with woman on top, aka Swooping Shakti
4. Side by side facing each other, aka Scissors
5. Man behind woman, aka Piercing Tiger

Regardless of how many positions you choose to do, the main credos of spiritual lovemaking hold for them all: This is a blending of mind, body, and spirit and your aim is connecting into oneness, not just getting off.

1. YAB YUM

In Yab Yum the spine is aligned with gravity, which is an essential ingredient for drawing energy to the higher chakras, or energy centers, and for stimulating the pineal and pitu-

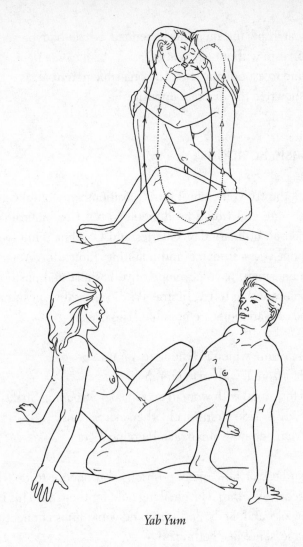

Yab Yum

itary gland, which is considered critical for enlightenment to occur. The partners sit erect and face-to-face. The woman is astride the man, who is cross-legged and supporting her weight on his thighs. Her legs are open and around him, with the soles of her feet touching. Note that the slight elevation of the woman brings her partner's chakras into alignment. If necessary, to alleviate the stress on the man's thighs, a pillow is used under the woman's hips.

According to Margot Anand, the Yab Yum position is "the ultimate form of Tantric union." In this position, the position of the man and woman allow the chakras, the energy centers, to be more aligned so that the energy can flow more easily up and down and through the partners.

Before going into formal Tantric practice, you may want to consider a more relaxed starting position such as in the lower illustration on page 220. It lets you find your comfort place, and you can initiate small pelvic rocking to build sensation before moving to the more connected illustration (shown at top of page 220).

2. HORIZONTAL WITH MAN ON TOP

According to the Taoists, the horizontal position (with the man on top), "respects the woman's innate nature—her

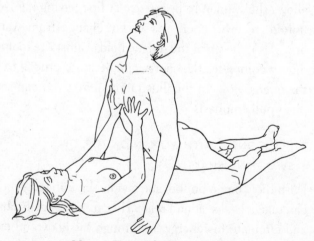

Man on Top, with Tongue Press

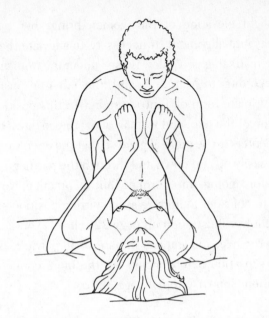

Push-Pull

qualities of water, coolness and slow rhythm. The posture allows the woman to be passive at first, giving her time to unfold, receive, open and slowly change from water to fire." Also, the tip of the tongue held against the roof of the mouth completes the energy circuit and is crucial to allow the energy flow. In the illustration above, you can see the push-pull emphasis.

3. HORIZONTAL WITH WOMAN ON TOP, OR SWOOPING SHAKTI

With the woman on top, she is now the initiator. The man can take a backseat and relax. He can more easily channel and circulate his energy up through his body and toward the woman. He is the one receiving and relaxing. The first

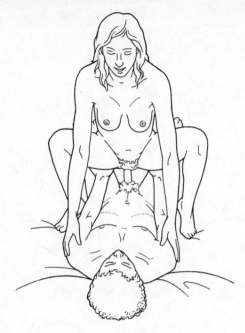

Swooping Shakti

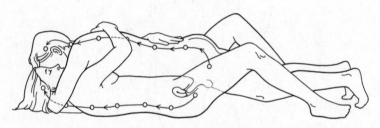

Circulating Sexual Energy

illustration (above) shows the woman in the ideal position to initiate her Pompoir power (i.e., Kegel exercise) on her lover. As I discuss later, this is crucial in creating the Wave of Bliss. The second variation illustrated above shows the energy circulating between the couple along the chakra pathway.

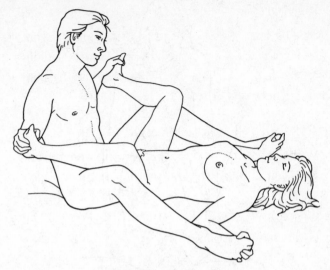

Completing the Circuit

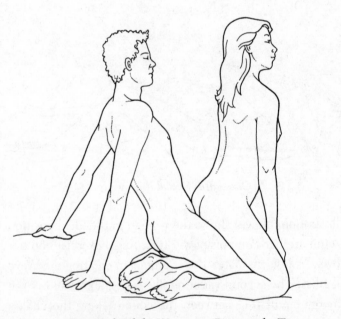

Man Behind the Woman, or Piercing the Tiger

4. COMPLETING THE CIRCUIT

Side by side, facing each other, the couple are completing and holding the energy circuits closed by holding each other's feet in their hands while maintaining connection and penetration.

5. THE MAN BEHIND THE WOMAN, OR PIERCING TIGER

With the man behind the woman, the woman can tighten her vaginal channel with the PC pump muscle (this is what the Kegels work) to heighten the sensation for both herself and her partner. Also, the tightness of entry between her thighs is good if a man is long and she is shallow.

The Techniques

As Kenneth Ray Stubbs, Ph.D., points out in his book *The Essential Tantra*, Tantra can be broken down into three essential ideas that should direct your approach:

➤ Time: Be present and let go of future expectations.
➤ Contact: Maintain contact with your partner at all times.
➤ Flow: Allow a natural flow from one movement to another, one moment of stillness and concentration to another.

If you keep these three concepts in mind as you begin to practice these techniques, you will greatly increase your ability to reach a spiritual or ecstatic state with your lover. Here are some other considerations to keep in mind before you choose a position. I've borrowed these steps from the wonderful Mantak Chia book *The Multi-Orgasmic Man*:

1. To harmonize and relax better with your partner, place similar body parts together: lips to lips, hands to hands, genitals to genitals.
2. To stimulate and excite each other, place dissimilar parts together: lips to ears, mouth to genitals, genitals to anus.
3. The person who is doing the most moving (generally the person on top) gives the most energy to the other partner. The person underneath can move as well to complement the movement of the person on top. This will help expand, circulate, and exchange sexual energy more quickly.

SECRET FROM LOU'S ARCHIVES

According to Charles and Caroline Muir, the potent kiss is a Tantric technique that uses an energetic conduit between the valley of a woman's upper lip and her clitoris. "The lover gently sucks on her upper lip, using his tongue and lips to draw in on the frenulum which stretches from the inside of the upper lip to the point on the gum directly above the two front teeth. As he sucks her upper lip, she sucks his lower lip and visualizes the subtle channel that runs from her frenulum to her clitoris. Once that channel opens as a conduit for sexual energy, a woman may be able to experience deep clitoral stimulation—even orgasm—from the kiss alone."

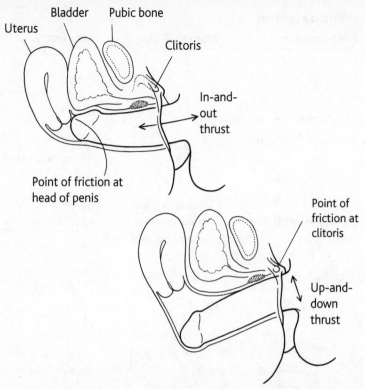

Bladder Pubic bone

Uterus

Clitoris

In-and-out thrust

Point of friction at head of penis

Point of friction at clitoris

Up-and-down thrust

Once the couple has decided the flow of a lovemaking session (you can make it either relaxing or exciting), then they can try the different techniques. In a general way, the approach to intercourse in a Tantric manner is about a shift in attitude: being open and relaxed and in touch with each other at a very deep, subtle level.

In terms of what you're actually doing, nothing is changing all that much. It's about where you consciously put the emphasis. For instance, the in-and-out thrust, in which the penis is thrust deeper into the woman, is the more vigorous style. You can make it more slow and gentle by literally slowing your thrust. The up-and-down thrust is more for the slow, relaxing

Woman's Feet on His Shoulders

Woman Riding

Rear Entry

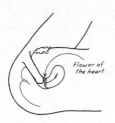

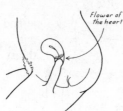

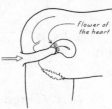

Deepest—
stimulates cervical
area

Woman moving
up and down—
deepest, cervical

Deepest—
straight in

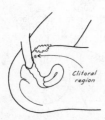

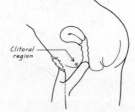

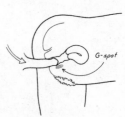

Man on tiptoe—
stimulates clitoris

Woman leaning
forward—clitoral

Man on tiptoe—
shallow G-spot

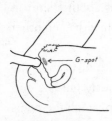

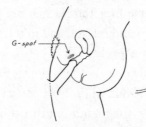

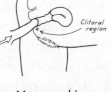

Man crouching—
stimulates G-spot
front wall

Woman leaning back
with up-and-down
action—G-spot

Man crouching—
shallow thrust—
clitoral

mood as the man will have to remain fairly close to the woman in order to maintain constant stimulating contact with the clitoral area. Keep this in mind as you move through the various techniques described below. In the illustrations opposite, you can observe the various techniques to easily adjust the stimulation area with one subtle position change.

THE KABAZZAH

Kabazzah, which is also known as Pompoir (by the French), Quivering Butterfly (Eastern), Kegels (by us North Americans), and Snapping Pussy (by some who prefer a flair), refers to the Eastern technique where the male partner is passive and the female uses only abdominal and vaginal muscle contractions to "milk" his penis. This is basically what I've described previously as a Kegel exercise, but used as a form of sexual expression, the move goes beyond strengthening and toning the PC muscles and becomes a technique a woman can use to stimulate her man's penis while he is inside of her.

While the woman moves her muscles, both partners should try to relax and enjoy the sensations of the union. Remember, this is slow, subtle sensation. The more in tune both of you are to the internal movement, the more stimulation can build and the more pleasure you will experience.

THE BIG DRAW

This technique as taught by Master Mantak Chia stems from a branch of Chinese medicine, which is popularly referred to as sexual kung fu. Its goal is to increase your orgasmic potential. This process takes learning and practice, so

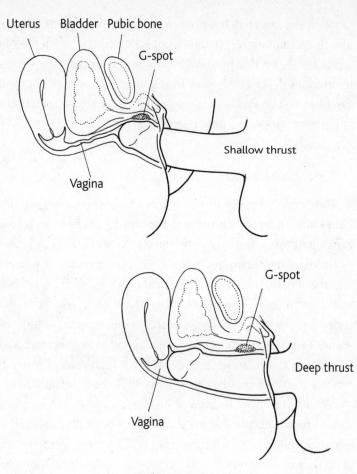

The Big Draw

don't be discouraged if you feel awkward or uncomfortable as you begin to test the waters. But believe me, the results are real and quite enjoyable—for both your lady and yourself.

In the Big Draw, the man practices stopping thrusting as he feels orgasm is imminent. When he feels he is about to come, he pulls out, to within an inch of withdrawing from the woman's vagina. The most important part of the move is the change in depth of thrusting. The man never totally withdraws so he maintains a vacuumlike feeling with his strong, deep penetrations. The Big Draw itself refers to the man's ability to move energy up through his body and use it to keep his PC muscles strong so he can control the emissions if he should choose to do so.

To enhance this technique one can use the Three Finger Draw. In this technique a man (or his partner) puts pressure on the mid-perineal area to stop ejaculation. This will help the man become familiar with the sensation of controlling ejaculation and learn how to know his timing more accurately. If his lover gets involved, this can also be a shared, intimate moment.

This is an important practice and must be done right. I would recommend reading Chia's *The Multi-Orgasmic Man* to familiarize oneself.

THE WAVE OF BLISS

The Wave of Bliss is a stunning technique that has the power to bring a couple together at the most intense, spiritual level. This is Margot Anand's favorite technique to use in the Yab Yum position, and I've used her description here because of its clarity and simplicity. You will both need a supportive cushion or pillow. According to Ms. Anand, there are seven essential steps:

1. PELVIC ROCKING

You begin by kneeling down on your cushions and facing each other, not touching. Gently move into a seated position, with your legs comfortably crossed. Close your eyes and focus on what is happening inside of your body and your heart. Begin to rock your pelvis forward and back, toward and away from each other, gently brushing your genitals and anus against the pillow. Do this for about five minutes and pay attention to the growing sensation in your genitals.

2. CULTIVATING AROUSAL

In this same position, keeping your eyes closed, continue the pelvic rocking and emphasize sensations in your genitals by squeezing your PC muscles (the Kegel exercise, as I describe in chapter 8). As you rock backward, tighten the genital muscles; as you rock forward, relax them. You are creating a sensual rhythm here that continues to build sensation and stimulation; in fact, you might feel a warmth and tingling in your genitals and pelvis.

3. OPENING THE INNER FLUTE TOGETHER

Now you are warm and ready to open your eyes and look at each other. Try synchronizing your rocking movements. Continue squeezing your PC muscles and being aware of your genital sensations. It's also important to maintain eye contact with each other so your connection stays alert and continues to deepen.

As you rock your pelvis backward and tighten your pelvic muscles, inhale deeply, imagining that you are pulling the sexual energy upward and out through the top of your head. As you rock your pelvis forward, relax the genital muscles and exhale, imagining the sexual energy moving back down through your body and out the genitals.

Stay in tune with each other as you breathe. Keep looking in each other's eyes, stay relaxed, and gradually let yourselves synchronize your rhythm. Try it fast, then try it

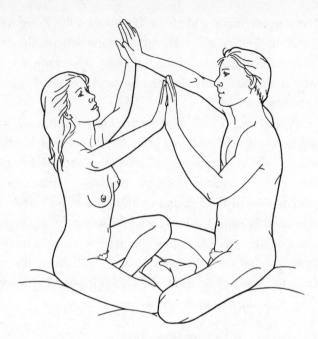

The Playful Wave

slow, playing with the pace that is right for you. Even though your lips are not touching, imagine that you are kissing each other through your breath.

4. THE PLAYFUL WAVE

This step requires some "dynamic dance music," suggests Anand. I would choose any kind of music that has a sensual, rhythmic beat that has an upbeat or playful tone. Maintain eye contact and remain seated on your cushions and turn on your music. Slowly reach out toward each other with your hands and touch your palms playfully, following the music as if your hands were dancing. Now you each bring your entire body into the dance, moving your arms, upper torso, and pelvis. Let your bodies move to the music and let your breath carry the movement. Be aware of who is leading and who is following, who is pushing and who is yielding. Then switch roles and feel the difference between the two.

Anand suggests introducing massage oil and gently massaging each other, sliding your hands over each other's skin. When you are ready, oil and caress each other's genitals, as you continue the slow, undulating movement of your bodies in the rocking rhythm. Then approach each other and "assume the position of the wave." In other words, the woman moves on top of the man, while he guides his penis ("vajra") into her vagina ("yoni"). Even if the man does not have an erection, he can still assume this position, pressing his penis against her.

5. CONNECTING BREATH TO BREATH

Now the woman wraps her legs around him, while he remains seated in a cross-legged position (this is called the Lotus Position). Feel free to use pillows to make the position more comfortable. Once you are both comfortable, take a few minutes to relax and feel each other's breath. Begin the gentle rocking again, along with the squeezing of the PC muscles. Move against each other and harmonize your rhythms.

When you are ready, begin to kiss and imagine that you are exchanging breath with your partner.

6. OPENING TO YOUR INNER LIGHT

At this point, you and your partner are becoming more and more aroused, nearing orgasmic sensations. As Anand says, "This step is key to moving orgasmic energy from the genitals and transforming it into an ecstatic and meditative experience." Continue kissing and exchanging breath. Close your eyes and let your eyes roll slightly upward and focus them on the Third Eye, that place in the center of your forehead, between your eyes. Tantrikas believe this is the seat of soul awareness. Draw all your sexual energy upward toward this point. Think of moving the sensation from your genital region through your pelvis, up through your belly, through your throat, and up through your Third Eye. Once you arrive at the Third Eye, hold your breath and keep squeezing your genital muscles. Now try to relax the rest of your body.

After a while, Anand states, "you may have the feeling of an explosion of light or a shooting star or fireworks." All along, continue kissing and exchanging breath. While you have been inhaling, your partner is exhaling, doing so very slowly and consciously, holding *your* breath as a way to slow *your* rhythm and accentuate the control of energy. Continue this exercise for several minutes and when you want to stop, bring your focus and energy down from the Third Eye to the genitals.

7. THE INFINITE CYCLE

In this final step, you stay locked within each other and continue breathing together. As the woman inhales and then exhales into her partner's mouth, she concentrates on moving the energy from her genitals up through her body and into her lover. The man receives her breath (when he inhales) and moves the energy down through his body out his vajra (penis) and into her yoni (vagina). This is a flow-

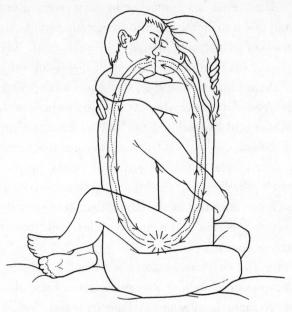

The Infinite Cycle

ing, rhythmic movement, different from step 6 above in that there is no holding of breath.

The intensity of this last step can lead to orgasm if either or both of you want to share that pleasure. You can also choose to relish in this wave of bliss that the rocking, breathing, kissing, and pure rhythm of sensation has created.

The Tantric Orgasm

You've waited, and waited, and now it's time. Here is the step-by-step description of achieving the ultimate orgasm, Tantra style. I've borrowed from the description that David Ramsdale uses in his book *Sexual Energy Ecstasy*. The road to orgasm begins with the man and woman in the Yab Yum position, with the man penetrating the woman.

1. The woman contracts her PC muscles while the man remains still, not moving his pelvis at all.
2. She is only squeezing her PC muscles, not moving her hips or pelvis.
3. You can caress and kiss and gaze into each other's eyes, but remain motionless below your hips.
4. Keep in mind that the woman is the actor or giver of energy in this exercise, and the man is the receiver and is therefore in a more passive role.
5. Maintain a calm, relaxed state of mind and body.
6. By this point, the man is responding to the woman's genital squeezing of his penis. Both of you are becoming highly aroused from the genital sensations.
7. After a while, this stimulation may become very intense and you might feel the urge to orgasm. The woman should back off the intensity of her squeezing so that the orgasm can be delayed.
8. After about fifteen minutes, Ramsdale says, you "will experience a bioelectrical force field effect." In other words, the sensations the two of you have created are so intense that you feel alone and separate from your surroundings, as if joined as one. This is an electric, transcendent feeling of bliss shared with your lover.
9. Stay with this feeling as long as you wish. Ramsdale recommends staying in the "electrical force field" another fifteen minutes in order to come to full Tantric orgasm. When you do choose to release

into the pleasure of orgasm, you may feel exuberant and expansive, transported to another level of consciousness—that is, a state of spiritual ecstasy.

Spiritual sex is by its nature a very personal, subtle experience. It taps into a deep reservoir of powerful emotion between two people, and when this emotion is expressed and shared between two people who love each other, they can transport themselves to another realm that has no other name than the spiritual.

This kind of experience may not be for everyone, but those with the curiosity to try it may discover new limits and potential for sexual pleasure, beyond what they had previously imagined. So enjoy!

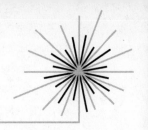

A Final Note

O ur sexuality is a mirror of our inner identity, that part of ourselves that makes us uniquely who we are. Some may call this the "soul," but I like to think of it simply as who we feel we are. This personality stamp comes out in all our interactions and relationships—especially our sexual relationships.

Since sex is the most intimate experience we can share with another human being, it makes sense that it exposes this inner identity of ours. How else can we be but honest when we make love? In my years of listening to men and women describe and discuss their sexual experiences, I've heard them talking straight from this inner, complicated, vulnerable place. All is revealed in a sexual relationship. And for this reason, it should be cherished, honored, and treated with the utmost respect.

Sexually Transmitted Diseases (STDs)

Chlamydia

Chlamydia is often called the silent STD because there are usually no symptoms until the disease is in an advanced state. Symptoms for men and women can be burning during urination, a strange discharge from the vagina or penis, pain in the lower abdomen, pain during sex, and, for women, bleeding between periods. An estimated 4 million new cases will be contracted in the United States this year alone. Chlamydia is spread through oral sex and intercourse.

In women, it can cause a bacterial infection deep within the fallopian tubes, causing chronic pain, tubular pregnancies, and infertility. Chlamydia can be passed from mother to child during birth, causing eye, ear, and lung infections in newborns. The good news is that chlamydia is easily cured with antibiotics, but it must be tested for specifically.

Gonorrhea

Also referred to as the clap, gonorrhea, like chlamydia, is a bacterial infection that often goes undetected in women until permanent damage has already occurred. In men, the symptoms can include a yellow puslike discharge from the penis, pain while urinating, the need to urinate often, and pain in the lower abdomen. This STD is highly contagious and can be spread through any contact with the penis, vulvar area, mouth, or anus, even without penetration. If left untreated, it can cause sterilization, tubular pregnancies, and chronic pain. It can also lead to pelvic inflammatory disease (PID). Gonorrhea can be passed from mother to child during birth, causing eye, ear, and lung infections.

Syphilis

Syphilis is a very dangerous bacterial infection, and an estimated 104,000 new cases in men and women will be contracted this year in the United States. If left untreated, syphilis can be fatal or cause irreparable damage to the heart, brain, eyes, and joints. Forty percent of all babies born to mothers with syphilis die during childbirth. Symptoms are painless sores, rashes on the palms and feet, and swollen lymph nodes. This disease is highly contagious through oral, vaginal, and anal sex, as well as through open wounds on the skin. When detected early, syphilis is curable with strong doses of antibiotics. Syphilis is common in heterosexual men in certain parts of the country and very rare in others.

Pelvic Inflammatory Disease (PID)

PID can affect women and is most often the result of advanced stages of chlamydia or gonorrhea. It is the leading cause of infertility in the United States. The most common symptom of PID is pain in the lower abdomen. Other symptoms include bleeding between periods, increased amount or changed vaginal discharge, nausea or vomiting, and fever with chills. When detected early PID is not life-threatening, but if there has been damage to the fallopian tubes before detection, the damage is often permanent.

Trichomoniasis (Trich)

A form of vaginitis in women, trich is caused by a germ that is spread through intercourse. An estimated 3 million new cases of vaginitis will be contracted in the United States this year. Not all forms of vaginitis are sexually transmitted, but the symptoms are similar. Yeast infections are a very common form of vaginitis not necessarily spread through sexual contact. A woman can get vaginitis by douching, taking antibiotics, wearing damp underwear, adhering to a poor diet, and by using vaginal products such as lubricants, sprays, and birth control devices. Symptoms can include discharge that is green, yellow, or gray with an unusual odor, itching in or around the vagina, and pain during sex and/or during urination. It is more uncomfortable than harmful. Vaginitis is easily treatable through a prescription medication and by some medications sold over the counter.

Herpes

It is estimated that somewhere between 200,000 and 500,000 new cases of genital herpes will be contracted this year, and 30 million Americans are infected already. Even more frightening is the number of people who are not aware of already being infected.

There are two viruses that cause genital herpes: herpes simplex 1, which occurs orally, and herpes simplex 2, which occurs genitally. Herpes simplex 1 is typically what we refer to as cold sores on, around, or inside the lips and mouth. The visible symptoms of herpes simplex 2 include painful and/or itchy bumps or blisters on the genital area, in men typically on the shaft of the penis at the end of the foreskin or near the head of the penis. In women, the outbreak occurs near or inside the vagina and/or rectum. Men can also get herpes near the anus even if they've never had anal intercourse. Sometimes herpes lesions first appear in areas related to the genitals by nerve endings but not actually on the genitals. In this case, the buttocks and thighs are common sites.

Herpes is highly contagious when physical contact is made during an outbreak, but it can also be contagious when the virus appears to lie dormant. This is because in most people with herpes, it can reactivate without symptoms. Lab studies have found that in cases in which a person feels that herpes is not active, 5 percent of the time evidence of the infectious virus can be found on the skin.

The first outbreak of genital herpes usually lasts between twelve and fourteen days, while subsequent outbreaks are shorter in duration (four to five days) and are milder. There is no cure for this virus, though the medications acyclovir, famciclovir, and valacyclovir have proven to be highly successful in both minimizing the symptoms of current outbreaks and suppressing future recurrences. What, precisely, determines a herpes recurrence has not been determined; however, studies indicate there is a strong association between herpes outbreaks and stress.

While the symptoms of the herpes virus can be very uncomfortable to those who have them, the real danger of this sexually transmitted disease is to an unborn child, or to an immune suppressed individual (with HIV or AIDS, for example). Newborn (neonatal) herpes is also a worry, but recent information shows that this is very unlikely in cases where the mother has herpes prior to becoming pregnant. It is most often transmitted to the infant during delivery and can cause painful blisters and damage to the eyes, brain, and internal organs of a newborn baby. One in six will not survive at all. The important point about neonatal herpes is that it is almost always caused by men. The woman at greatest risk for giving birth to an affected baby experiences her transmission and first herpes episode late in pregnancy. Therefore, if you and your partner are working on getting pregnant, and the man has herpes and the woman does not, it is paramount for you to use proper safe-sex practices during pregnancy and consider suppressive antiviral treatment.

The good news is that when knowledge of genital herpes exists, a cesarean delivery can generally prevent damage to the child. In fact, the risk is so low these days that women who are having recurrent herpes episodes are only given a cesarean section if there is an active symptomatic lesion present.

If you think you have been exposed to herpes, there is only one test, a blood test called the Western blot, which can make this diagnosis without symptoms. Doctors more often perform viral culture tests by swabbing a lesion when it is in a very early stage of blistering or erosions.

Human Papilloma Virus (HPV)

The human papilloma virus, also known as condyloma, represents a family of viruses consisting of over 170 different types. There will be an estimated 1 million new cases of HPV diagnosed this year. Certain forms of HPV cause visible genital warts, though some strains of HPV infection cause no warts at all. Genital warts are growths that appear on the vulva, in or around the vagina or anus, on the cervix, and on the penis, scrotum, groin, or thigh. They can be raised or flat, single or multiple, small or large. All sexually active men and women are susceptible to contracting HPV. It is spread by direct contact during vaginal, oral, and anal sex with someone who has the virus. Though rare, infants can also be infected during childbirth. Besides being painful, certain strains of HPV can cause cervical cancer. The strains that cause genital warts, however, are not the strains associated with cervical cancer. (Only the physician can sort this out.) It is a virus that can lie dormant for years, and there is no known cure for this disease. Genital warts can be treated in several ways including freezing, laser surgery, chemical peels, and topical creams. The strains of HPV that don't produce genital warts usually go undetected until there is an abnormality in your Pap smear. Genital HPV is manageable with proper diagnosis. Men should look for testicular abnormalities, for example. Women should get regular Pap smears, and look for any new growths on the skin, which, even if painless, should be checked out.

Hepatitis B

An infection caused by the hepatitis B virus is usually not considered an STD; however, it is spread through infected semen, vaginal secretions, and saliva, and it can be passed from mother to child at the time of birth. You can also get it by direct contact with an infected person through open sores and cuts. If someone in your home is infected, you can contract hepatitis B by using the same razor or toothbrush.

However, this may not be as risky as it sounds. Studies have shown that <1 percent of household contacts become infected with the virus even if they live with someone who has chronic hepatitis B. Since the most prevalent way that hepatitis B is spread is through contaminated blood or blood products, 70 percent of all infections are in high-risk groups: IV drug abusers, homosexuals, and hemophiliacs. In 1996, there were only 10,637 reported cases in the United States.

Hepatitis B attacks the liver. In its mildest form, more than 50 percent develop no symptoms when exposed and 30 percent only develop flulike symptoms. In both cases, there is a 100 percent recovery and you have lifetime immunity to the virus. Approximately 20 percent of the time, you may develop enough symptoms to warrant an evaluation by your doctor, resulting in the diagnosis of hepatitis B infection.

However, 95 percent of those people that are diagnosed with hepatitis B recover fully and have lifetime immunity. Therefore, less than 5 percent of people that contract the illness become chronic carriers, and only 1.25 percent may proceed to cirrhosis and liver cancer fifteen to thirty years after the infection. Symptoms can be very much like those of the stomach flu. See your doctor immediately if you have nausea, unexplainable tiredness, dark urine, and/or yellowing of the eyes and skin. There are multiple medications on the market for hepatitis B, but most cause significant side effects. The most effective treatment for the infection is rest and a high-protein, high-carbohydrate diet.

There is a vaccination for hepatitis B. It is a series of shots, given in the arm. However, there are a growing number of significant side effects being reported from the vaccine, including arthritis, a plethora of neurological disorders, and chronic fatigue. You would be wise to practice safe sex with your partner—and both be tested for hepatitis B—rather than depending on the vaccine as "protection."

HIV / AIDS

Acquired immune deficiency syndrome (AIDS) is a diagnosis resulting from infection with the human immunodeficiency virus (HIV). Testing positive for HIV indicates an immune response resulting from exposure to HIV. HIV and AIDS are not the same thing, but one is the precursor of the other. You cannot get AIDS without having HIV, though you can be HIV positive without having an AIDS diagnosis. HIV attacks the immune system, leaving the body unable to fight off common sicknesses or other diseases. An estimated 45,000 people in the United States will contract the virus this year. It is a sexually infectious disease spread through blood, semen, and vaginal fluids. Touching, kissing, sharing food, coughing, mosquito bites, using common toilet seats, swimming in pools, and donating blood do *not* spread HIV. This is not an airborne virus and cannot be spread by casual contact. There are usually no symptoms accompanying HIV. People can get the virus and feel terrific for many years. Unfortunately, the virus almost always leads to AIDS eventually, and because the immune system fails, the symptoms for AIDS can look like anything from a cold to cancer. Although there is no cure for AIDS, there are new drugs that dramatically slow down HIV's effect on the immune system. Every sexually active man and woman should have an HIV test and wait the six months required to ensure a clean bill of health before having unprotected sex with any new exclusive partner.

There is a new HIV test, called OraSure, an oral specimen device that requires no blood collection and is 99 percent accurate. Like a blood test, it tests for the presence of HIV antibodies. Dr. Penelope Hitchcock at the National Institutes of Health (NIH) says that OraSure is a great product and that NIH has worked with the manufacturer.

While I've discussed the most common of the sexually transmitted diseases, there are more than fifty known STDs to date. Providing you with knowledge about them is not meant to scare you, but rather to empower you. No one should be frightened to take control of his or her sexual health. With this information, I hope being safe becomes a matter of mutual respect for you and your partner.

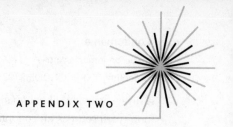

Resources

Where You Can Get the Toys

In collecting the best sources for toy products, I asked store owners several questions in order to verify their commitment to high quality and an open, encouraging attitude: Did they have a positive sex attitude? Would a woman be comfortable going into the store by herself or ordering over the phone? How big was its selection? Did they sell their mailing list? Was their e-mail site secure?

Catalogs are a great, safe way to introduce tools into the relationship. The very act of choosing a toy can be a bonding, intimate experience. It's a gentle way to suggest what you'd like to try. By looking at the pictures together, you and your partner can feel each other out about what may seem like fun, what may seem too risky, and so on. Initially, making suggestions can make you and her feel vulnerable. Women especially fear being rejected. Remember, gentlemen, they don't want to risk being perceived as "loose," if they suggest using a sex toy.

Essentially, the catalogs I am recommending are tasteful. A couple of these outfits are more oriented toward women, provide wonderful support staff to answer questions via an 800 number, and have careful explanations in the catalogs themselves. Other catalogs are a bit more edgy and less pristine. (Be aware, Adam & Eve sells their mailing list.)

Condomania

www.condomania.com

Order line: 800-9CONDOMS (926-6366)

This website and phone/mail order service is one of the best non-retail sources for condoms. Has a ROAD TEST chart on the site based on published articles. They offer a selection of over three hundred different condoms. The e-mail site uses SSL encryption when placing an order.

WEST COAST

SEATTLE

Toys in Babeland

707 East Pike St., Seattle WA 98122

206-328-2914 / Catalog: 800-658-9119

E-mail: biglove@babeland.com / Website: babeland.com

This is a female-run store, originally created as a place for women and their comfort. It now carries some male-oriented products. Workshops and seminars.

SAN FRANCISCO

Good Vibrations

Retail stores:

    1210 Valencia St., San Francisco CA 94110

    2502 San Pablo Ave., Berkeley CA 94702

Mail order:

    938 Howard St., Suite 101, San Francisco CA 94103

    415-974-8990 / 800-289-8423 (in the U.S.)

    Fax: 415-974-8989 / E-mail: goodvibe@well.com

    Website: http://www.goodvibes.com

Good Vibrations is one of the best all-around store/catalog combinations. Their specialty is vibrators—and they have an endless supply and selection. They also offer a vast array of lubricants, special massage oils, and videos and books. The selection of toys and leather goods is also of high quality, durability, and inventive styling. All their products have passed customer satisfaction tests. The staff is known for its courteous, nonjudgmental, sex-positive attitude, offering sensitive, knowledgeable, and helpful service.

LOS ANGELES

The Pleasure Chest

7733 Santa Monica Blvd., Los Angeles CA 90046
323-650-1022 / Order line: 800-753-4536
Fax: 323-650-1176 / Website: www.thepleasurechest.com

This Pleasure Chest targets a primarily gay male clientele, with a strong leather focus, though straight men and women will find many products for them, including videos and apparel.

Glow

8358½ West 3rd St., Los Angeles CA 90048
323-782-9080 / E-mail: glowspotLA@aol.com

Glow offers an outstanding selection of aromatherapy products. Custom blending available.

The Love Boutique

18637 Ventura Blvd., Tarzana CA 91356
818-342-2400
2924 Wilshire Blvd., Santa Monica CA 90403
310-453-3459 / Toll-free ordering: 888-568-4663

The two stores are female owned and operated and are open seven days a week. While they offer a small selection of items, the customer is treated with care by a knowledgeable staff. The staff seems uniquely focused on making women feel more at ease and comfortable with their sexuality.

Paradise Specialties
7344 Center Ave,. Huntington Beach, CA 92647

714-898-0400

Refined comfortable environment.

SAN DIEGO

F Street Stores (ten stores in the San Diego area)
751 Fourth Ave., San Diego CA 92101 / 619-236-0841

2004 University Ave., San Diego CA 92104 / 619-298-2644

7998 Miramar Rd., San Diego CA 92126 / 619-549-8014

1141 Third Ave., Chula Vista CA 92011 / 619-585-3314

237 East Grand, Escondido CA 92023 / 619-480-6031

The stores in this chain offer a wide range of male and female products; it was also one of the first to create a women's novelty section.

Condoms Plus
1220 University Ave., San Diego CA 92103

619-291-7400

This is a store "with a woman in mind." It is a general license store for all sorts of gifts, as well as condoms. In other words, you can buy a stuffed animal for your child as well as an adult novelty item for your husband. The novelties, however, are in their own section of the store.

MIDWEST

CHICAGO

The Pleasure Chest (affiliated with the store in New York)
3155 North Broadway, Chicago IL 60657

773-525-7152 / Catalog sales: 800-316-9222

The majority of customers are women and couples. This is the store that defined what an adult store should be like: clean, bright, tastefully presented, with nonjudgmental salespeople who look like you and me. This and the New York store (see page 252) show the impact of being run and operated by the owner, who focuses on taking good care of the customer.

Frenchy's
872 North State St., Chicago IL 60611
312-337-9190

This store has undergone a major renovation in appearance and size. It is now three times larger and offers a range of products for men and women.

MINNEAPOLIS/ST. PAUL

Fantasy House Gifts
716 West Lake Street, Minneapolis MN 55408
612-824-2459 / Website: www.fantasygifts.com

There are eight Fantasy House stores in the area, including Bloomington, Bernsville, St. Louis Park, Crystal, Fridley, Coon Rapids, and St. Paul—and two stores in New Jersey, Marlton and Turnersville. Adult material and novelties presented with a comfortable Midwestern environment and attitude. They recently added the Condom Kingdom store in Minneapolis to their operation.

OKLAHOMA

Christies Toy Box
1184 North MacArthur Blvd., Oklahoma City OK 73127
405-942-4622

Christies is part of a chain of adult stores, ranked number one in the state of Oklahoma; stores also exist in Texas.

A Woman's Touch

600 Williamson St., Madison WI, 53703

888-621-8880 or 608-250-1928 / Website: www.touchofawoman.com

Newsletter posted on site with seminars and workshops. Prescreened books and videos so that they are female friendly. Site encrypted. Run by an M.D. and M.S.W. (social worker) and therefore very current information updates.

EAST COAST

NEW YORK

The Pleasure Chest

156 Seventh Ave. South (between Charles and Perry),
New York NY 10014

212-242-4185 / Catalog sales: 800-316-9222

New York store customer service: 800-643-1025

E-mail: apleasurechest.com / Website: apleasurechest.com

The New York store and its Chicago sister store are both popular, classy, and well stocked, with a range of products for both men and women, straight and gay.

Eve's Garden

119 West 57th St., Suite 1201, New York NY 10019

212-757-8651 / Orders: 800-848-3837

Website: www.evesgarden.com

This is a female-owned and -operated store. What the Pleasure Chest did in 1972 for gay male consumers Eve's Garden did for women in 1974. Located in the heart of midtown Manhattan, Eve's Garden is in the least likely of areas. It is known far and wide as the matriarch of feminine-focused, sex-positive merchandising.

Toys in Babeland

94 Rivington St., New York NY 10002

212-375-1701 / E-mail: comments@babeland.com

Website: www.babeland.com

THE SOUTH

NORTH CAROLINA

Adam & Eve

PO Box 800, North Carrboro NC 27510

800-765-ADAM (2326) / Customer service: 919-644-1212

This is the biggest mail-order adult products company in the United States. It offers a full range of products.

TEXAS

Forbidden Fruit

108 E. North Loop Blvd., Austin, TX 78751

512-453-8090 / Website: www.forbiddenfruit.com

Three locations in Austin. Very female friendly atmosphere. Seminars. The site is secure.

CANADA

BRITISH COLUMBIA

Womyn's Ware Inc.

896 Commercial Drive, Vancouver, British Columbia V5L 3Y5

888-996-9273, order desk; 604-254-2543, store.

Website: www.womynsware.com

CALGARY

The Love Boutique

9737 MacLeod Trail S., Calgary, AB T2J 0P6

403-252-1846

Just For Lovers
Store #1: 920 36th St. NE, #114 / 403-273-6242
Store #2: 4014 MacLeod Trail S. / 403-243-2554
Store #3: 1415 17th Ave. SW / 403-245-9505
Store #4: 3630 Brentwood Rd. NW, #515 / 403-282-7125

NOVA SCOTIA

Venus Envy
1598 Barrington St., Halifax, Nova Scotia B3J 1Z6
902-422-0004 / Website: www.venusenvy.ca

ONTARIO

Venus Envy
110 Parent Ave., Ottawa, Ontario K1N 7B4
613-789-4646 / Website: www.venusenvy.ca

TORONTO

Seduction
577 Yonge St., Toronto, ON M4Y 1Z2
416-966-6969

This recently opened retail operation is the largest adult novelty store in North America, measuring 15,000 square feet on three floors. The customers are well taken care of by young, fresh-faced college women who know what they are selling.

Come As You Are
701 Queen Street West, Toronto, ON M6J 1E6
877-504-7934 / Website: www.comeasyouare.com

"Good sex is a cooperative effort." Only cooperative-run sex store in Canada.

VANCOUVER

Love Nest

161 East 1st St., North Vancouver, BC V7L 1B2

604-987-1175 / Website: lovenest.ca

As we are going to press, Tony and Kira, the husband/wife owner-operators, were just opening their second store in Whistler, BC.

Any of the listed products in the book can be purchased through The Sexuality Seminars/FRANKLY SPEAKING, INC. All transactions are confidential and we do not sell our mailing list. To purchase products, inquire about Lou Paget's seminar schedule, book a seminar, be placed on the FRANKLY SPEAKING mailing list, or to get more information, call 1-877-SexSeminars (1-877-739-7364).

Purchases can be made by Visa/MasterCard, cash, or check. FRANKLY SPEAKING, INC. shows on all bank statements and is the name under which all correspondence is sent. All product is discreetly packaged and shipped Priority Post unless otherwise requested. The Speciality Sophist-Kits™ gift boxes can arrive in presentation style (open) or closed—for a bigger surprise. They are delivered UPS or Federal Express and are shipped through Artfull Baskets.

For more information, we can reached at:

Frankly Speaking, Inc.

11601 Wilshire Blvd., Suite 500, Los Angeles CA 90025

310-556-3623

E-mail: LouPaget@aol.com / Website: LouPaget.com

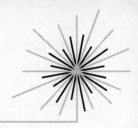

Bibliography

Anand, Margot. *The Art of Sexual Ecstasy: The Path of Sacred Sexuality for Western Lovers.* Jeremy Tarcher, Los Angeles. 1989.

Anand, Margot. *The Art of Sexual Magic: Cultivating Sexual Energy to Transform Your Life.* Tarcher/Putnam, New York. 1995.

Anand, Margot. *Sexual Ecstasy: The Art of Orgasm. Exercises from the Art of Sexual Magic.* Tarcher/Putnam, New York. 2000.

Bakos, Susan Crain. *What Men Really Want: Straight Talk from Men about Sex.* St. Martin's, New York. 1990.

Barbach, Lonnie. *For Each Other: Sharing Sexual Intimacy.* Anchor Press/Doubleday, New York. 1982.

Bechtel, Stefan. *The Practical Encyclopedia of Sex and Health.* Rodale, Emmaus, Pa. 1993.

Bechtel, Stefan. *Sex: A Man's Guide.* Rodale, Emmaus, Pa. 1996.

Bell, Simon, Richard Curtis, and Helen Fielding. *Who's Had Who.* Warner Books, New York. 1990.

Birch, Robert. *Oral Caress: The Loving Guide to Exciting a Woman. A Comprehensive Illustrated Manual on the Joyful Art of Cunnilingus.* PEC Publications, Columbus, Ohio. 1996.

Bishop, Clifford. *Sex and Spirit: Ecstasy and Transcendence Ritual and Taboo. The Undivided Self.* Little, Brown and Company, New York. 1996.

Blank, Joani. *Good Vibrations: The Complete Guide to Vibrators.* Down There Press, San Francisco. 1989.

Block, Joel D., and Susan Crain Bakos. *Sex Over 50.* Rewar Books, Paramus N.J. 1999.

Boteach, Shumley. *Kosher Sex: A Recipe for Passion and Intimacy.* Main Street Books, Doubleday, New York. 1999.

Brame, Gloria. *Come Hither: A Commonsense Guide to Kinky Sex.* Fireside Books, New York. 1999.

Caine, K. Winston. *The Male Body: An Owner's Manual*. Rodale, Emmaus, Pa. 1996.

Chalker, Rebecca. *The Clitoral Truth: The Secret World at Your Fingertips*. Seven Stories Press, New York. 2000.

Chang, Dr. Stephen T. *The Tao of Sexology: The Book of Infinite Wisdom*. Tao Publishing, Reno, Nevada. 1986.

Chesser, Eustace. *Strange Loves: The Human Aspects of Sexual Deprivation*. William Morrow and Company, New York. 1971.

Chia, Mantak and Douglas Abrams. *The Multi-Orgasmic Man: How Every Man Can Experience Multiple Orgasms and Dramatically Enhance His Sexual Relationship*. Harper, San Francisco. 1997.

Chia, Mantak and Maneewan Chia. *Healing Love through the Tao: Cultivating Female Sexual Energy*. Healing Tao Books, Huntington, New York. 1986.

Chia, Mantak and Michael Winn. *Taoist Secrets of Love: Cultivating Male Sexual Energy*. Aurora Press, Santa Fe. 1984.

Chichester, B., ed. *Sex Secrets: Ways to Satisfy Your Partner Every Time*. Rodale, Emmaus, Pa. 1996.

Chu, Valentin. *The Yin-Yang Butterfly: Ancient Chinese Sexual Secrets for Western Lovers*. Tarcher/Putnam, New York. 1993.

Cohen, Angela and Sarah Gardner Fox. *The Wise Woman's Guide to Erotic Videos: 300 Sexy Videos for Every Woman—and Her Lover*. Broadway Books, New York. 1997.

Comfort, Alex. *The Joy of Sex: A Gourmet Guide to Love Making*. Fireside/Simon & Schuster, New York. 1972.

Comfort, Alex. *The New Joy of Sex: A Gourmet Guide to Lovemaking for the Nineties*. Crown, New York. 1991.

Danielou, Alain. *The Complete Kama Sutra: The First Unabridged Modern Translation of the Classic Indian Text*. Park Street Press, Rochester, Vt. 1994.

Deida, David. *The Way of the Superior Lover: A Spiritual Guide to Sexual Skills*. Plexus, Austin, Tex. 1997.

Dodson, Betty. *Sex for One. The Joy of Selfloving*. Crown, New York. 1996.

Douglas, Nik, and Penny Slinger. *Sexual Secrets: The Alchemy of Ecstasy; 10th Anniversary Issue*. Destiny Books, Rochester, Vt. 1989.

Eichel, Edward and Philip Nobile. *The Perfect Fit: How to Achieve Mutual Fulfillment and Monogamous Passion through the New Intercourse*. Signet, New York. 1993.

Ellison, Carol Rinkleib. *Women's Sexualities: Generations of Women Share Intimate Secrets of Sexual Self-Acceptance*. New Harbinger, Oakland, Calif. 2000.

Fisher, Helen. *Anatomy of Love; The Natural History of Monogamy, Adultery and Divorce*. W. W. Norton, New York. 1992.

Fisher, Helen. *The First Sex: The Natural Talents of Women and How They Are Changing the World*. Random House, New York. 1999.

George, Stephen C. *A Lifetime of Sex: The Ultimate Manual on Sex, Women and Relationships for Every Stage of a Man's Life*. Rodale, Emmaus, Pa. 1998.

Goldstein, Irwin and Larry Rothstein. *The Potent Male*. Regenesis CyclePress, (no city given). 1995.

Hatcher, Robert A. *Contraceptive Technology*, 16th ed. Irvington Publishers, New York. 1994.

Hite, Shere. *The Hite Report: A Nationwide Study on Female Sexuality*. Dell, New York. 1976.

Hite, Shere. *The Hite Report: On Male Sexuality*. Ballantine, New York. 1981.

Holstein, M.D., Lana L. *How to Have Magnificent Sex: The Seven Dimensions of a Vital Sexual Connection*. Crown, New York. 2001.

Janus, Samuel and Cynthia Janus. *The Janus Report on Sexual Behavior: The First Broad-Scale Scientific National Survey Since Kinsey*. John Wiley & Sons, New York. 1993.

Kahn, Sandra. *The Kahn Report on Sexual Preferences*. Avon, New York. 1981.

Kaplan, Helen Singer. *The New Sex Therapy: The Active Treatment of Sexual Disorders*. Brunner/Mazel, New York. 1974.

Keesling, Barbara. *How to Make Love All Night (and Drive a Woman Wild). Male Multiple Orgasm and Other Secrets for Prolonging Lovemaking*. Harper Perennial, New York. 1994.

Keesling, Barbara. *Sexual Pleasure: Reaching New Heights of Sexual Arousal & Intimacy*. Hunter House, Alameda, Calif. 1993.

Kline-Graber, Georgia and Benjamin Graber. *Woman's Orgasm: A Guide to Sexual Satisfaction*. Popular Library, New York. 1976.

Kronhausen, Phyllis and Eberhard Kronhausen. *The Complete Book of Erotic Art*, vols. 1 and 2. Bell Publishing, New York. 1978.

Knutila, John. *Fit for Sex: A Man's Guide to Enhancing and Maintaining Peak Sexual Performance*. Reward Books, Paramus, N.J. 2000.

Ladas Kahn, Alice, Beverly Whipple, and John Perry. *The G-Spot: and Other Recent Discoveries about Human Sexual*. Dell, New York. 1982.

Legman, G. *The Intimate Kiss: The Modern Classic of Oral Erotic Technique*. Warner, New York. 1973.

Love, Brenda. *Encyclopedia of Unusual Sex Practices*. Barricade Books, New York. 1992.

Mann, A. T., Jane Lyle. *Sacred Sexuality*. Element Books Limited, Shaftsbury, Dorset, England. 1995.

Massey, Doreen. *Lovers' Guide Encyclopedia: The Definitive Guide to Sex and You*. Thunder's Mouth Press, New York. 1996.

Masters, William, Virginia Johnson, and Robert C. Kolodny. *Heterosexuality*. HarperCollins, New York. 1994.

Masters, William, and Virginia Johnson. *Human Sexual Response*. Little, Brown and Company, Boston. 1966.

McCutcheon, Marc. *The Compass in Your Nose and other Astonishing Facts about Humans*. Jeremy P. Tarcher, Los Angeles. 1989.

McCary, James Leslie. *Sexual Myths & Fallacies*. Schocken, New York. 1973.

Meletis, Chris D. *Better Sex Naturally: Herbs and Other Natural Supplements That Can Jump Start Your Sex Life*. The Philip Lief Group, (no city given). 2000.

Milsten, Richard and Julian Slowinski. *The Sexual Male: Problems and Solutions: A Complete Medical and Psychological Guide to Lifelong Potency*. W. W. Norton and Company, New York. 1999.

Mooney, Shane. *Useless Sexual Trivia: Tastefully Purient Facts about Everyone's Favorite Subject*. Fireside, New York. 2000.

Muir, Charles and Caroline Muir. *Tantra: The Art of Conscious Loving*. Mercury House, San Francisco. 1989.

Neret, Gilles. *Erotica Universalis*. Benedikt Taschen, Verlag, Germany. 1994.

O'Connell, Helen E., et al. "Anatomical Relationship Between the Urethra and Clitoris." *Journal of Urology* 159 (1998): 1892.

Ogden, Gina. *Women Who Love Sex: An Inquiry into the Expanding Spirit of Women's Erotic Experience*. Womanspirit Press, Cambridge, Mass. 1999.

Otto, Herbert A. *Liberated Orgasms: The Orgasmic Revolution*. Liberating Creations, Inc. Silverado, Calif. 1999.

Oxford English Dictionary, Second edition. Oxford University Press, Oxford. 1989.

Panati, Charles. *Sexy Origins and Intimate Things: The Rites and Rituals of Straights, Gays, Bi's, Drags, Trans, Virgins and Others*. Penguin Books, New York. 1998.

Parsons, Alexandra. *Facts & Phalluses: A Collection of Bizarre and Intriguing Truths, Legends and Measurements*. St. Martin's, New York. 1989.

Purvis, Kenneth. *The Male Sexual Machine: An Owner's Manual*. St. Martin's, New York. 1992.

Ramsdale, David and Ellen Ramsdale. *Sexual Energy Ecstasy. A Practical Guide to Lovemaking Secrets of the East and West*. Bantam, New York. 1993.

Rancier, Lance. *The Sex Chronicles: Strange-But-True Tales from Around the World*. General Publishing Group, Los Angeles. 1997.

Reinisch, Judith. *The Kinsey Institute New Report on Sex: What You Must Know to Be Sexually Literate*. St. Martin's, New York. 1990.

Rilly, Cheryl. *Great Moments in Sex*. Three Rivers Press, New York. 1999.

Sacks, Stephen. *The Truth About Herpes*, 4th ed. Gordon Soules Publishers, Vancouver, Canada. 1997.

Schwartz, Bob, and Leah Schwartz. *The One Hour Orgasm: How to Learn the Amazing "Venus Butterfly."* 3rd ed. Breakthru Publishing, Houston. 1999.

Smith, David, and Mike Gordon. *Strange but True Facts about Sex: The Illustrated Book of Sexual Trivia*. Meadowbook Press, Minn. 1989.

Smith, Richard. *The Dieter's Guide to Weight Loss During Sex*. Workman Publishing, New York. 1978.

Stoppard, Miriam. *The Magic of Sex: The Book That Really Tells Men about Women and Women about Men*. Dorling Kindersley, New York. 1991.

Stubbs, Kenneth Ray, and Louise-Andrée Saulnier. *Erotic Massage: The Touch of Love*. Secret Garden, Larkspur, Calif. 1993.

Taormino, Tristan. *The Ultimate Guide to Anal Sex for Women*. Cleis Press, San Francisco. 1998.

Tannahill, Reay. *Sex in History*. Scarborough House, Briarcliff Manor, New York. 1980.

Tannen, Deborah. *You Just Don't Understand: Women and Men in Conversation*. William Morrow, New York. 1990.

Taylor, Timothy. *The Prehistory of Sex: Four Million Years of Human Sexual Culture*. Bantam, New York. 1996.

Tepper, Mitchell Steven. "Attitudes, Beliefs, and Cognitive Process That May Impede or Facilitate Sexual Pleasure and Orgasm in People with Spinal Cord Injury." *Dissertation in Education*. Presented to the Faculties of the University of Pennsylvania in Partial Fulfillment of the Requirements for the Doctorate of Philosophy. 1999.

Tuleja, Tad. *Curious Customs: The Stories Behind 296 Popular American Rituals*. Harmony Books/Crown, New York. 1987.

Walker, Barbara G. *The Woman's Encyclopedia of Myths And Secrets*. Harper & Row, New York. 1983.

Walker, Morton. *Foods for Fabulous Sex: Natural Sexual Nutrients to Trigger Passion, Heighten Response, Improve Performance & Overcome Dysfunction*. Magni Group, McKinney, Tex. 1992.

Wallace, Irving. *The Nympho and Other Maniacs: The Lives, the Loves and the Sexual Adventures of Some Scandalous and Liberated Ladies*. Simon & Schuster, New York. 1971.

Watson, Cynthia Mervis. *Love Potions: A Guide to Aphrodisiacs and Sexual Pleasures*. Tarcher/Putnam, New York. 1993.

Welch, Leslee. *Sex Facts: A Handbook for the Carnally Curious*. Carol Publishing, New York. 1992.

Wildwood, Chrissie. *Erotic Aromatherapy: Essential Oils for Lovers*. Sterling, New York. 1994.

Worwood, Valerie Ann. *Scents & Scentuality: Aromatherapy & Essential Oils for Romance, Love and Sex*. New World Library, Novato, Calif. 1999.

Zacks, Richard. *History Laid Bare: Lover Perversity from the Ancient Etruscans to Warren G. Harding*. HarperCollins, New York. 1994.

Zilbergeld, Bernie. *Male Sexuality*. Bantam, New York. 1978.

Zilbergeld, Bernie. *The New Male Sexuality: The Truth about Men, Sex, and Pleasure*, Rev. edition. Bantam, New York. 1999.

Zimet, Susan and Victor Goodman. *The Great Cover-Up: A Condom Compendium*. Civan, Inc., New York. 1988.

Zimmerman, Jack, and Jaquelyn McCandless. *Flesh and Spirit: The Mystery of the Intimate Relationship*. Bramble Books, Las Vegas. 1998.